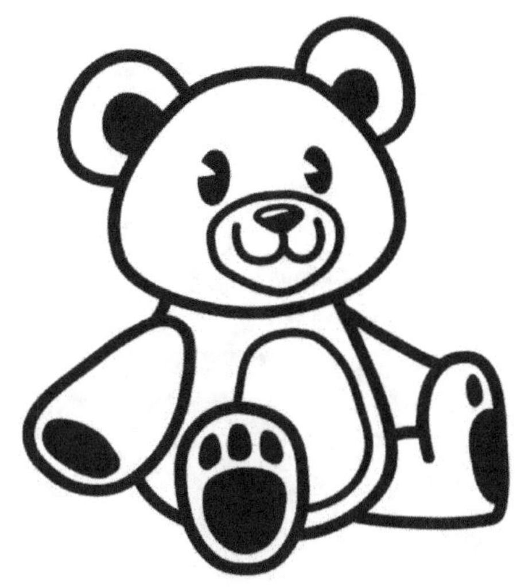
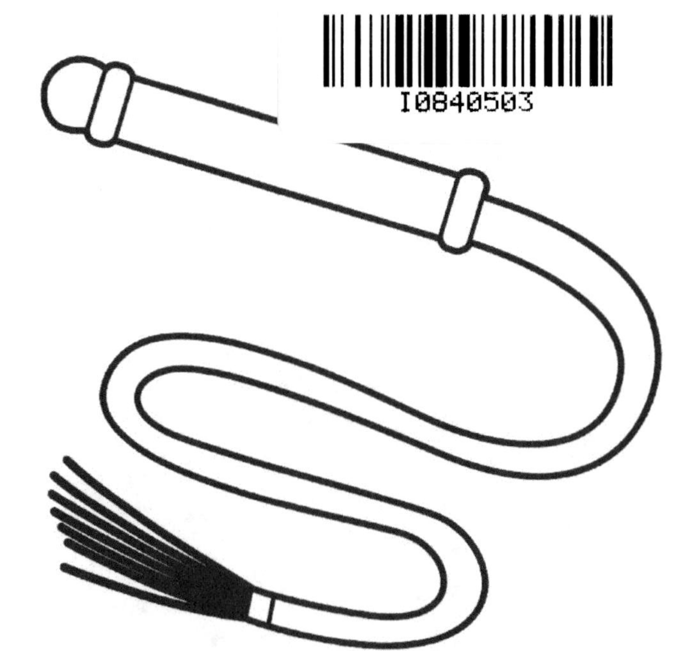

This Book Belongs To

____

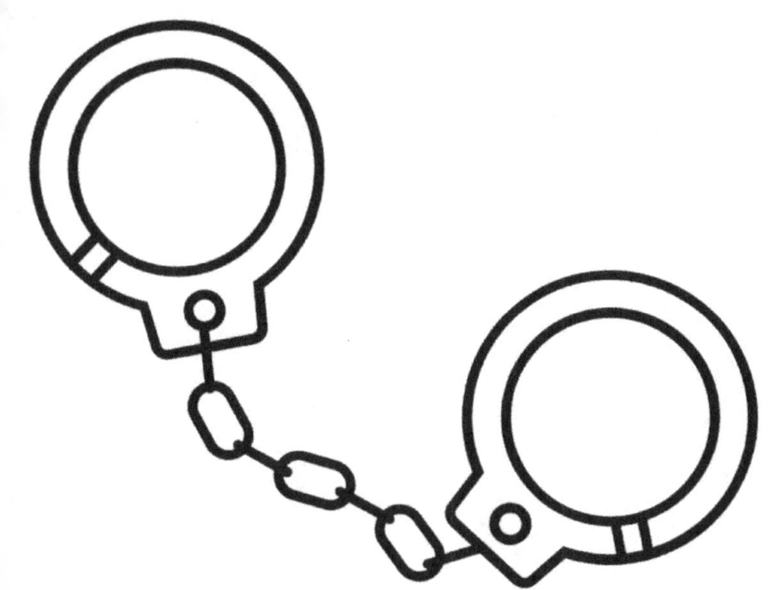
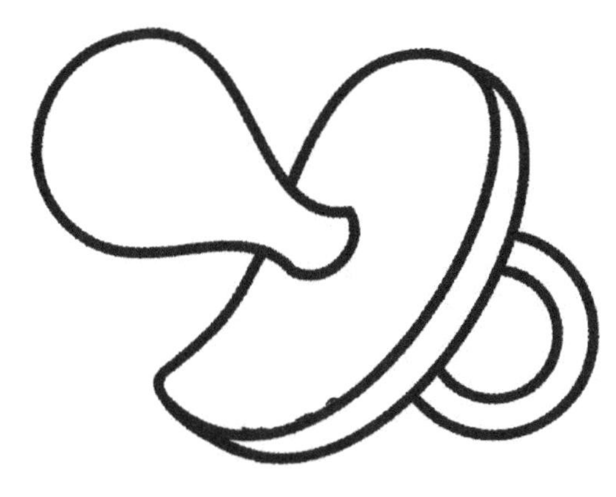

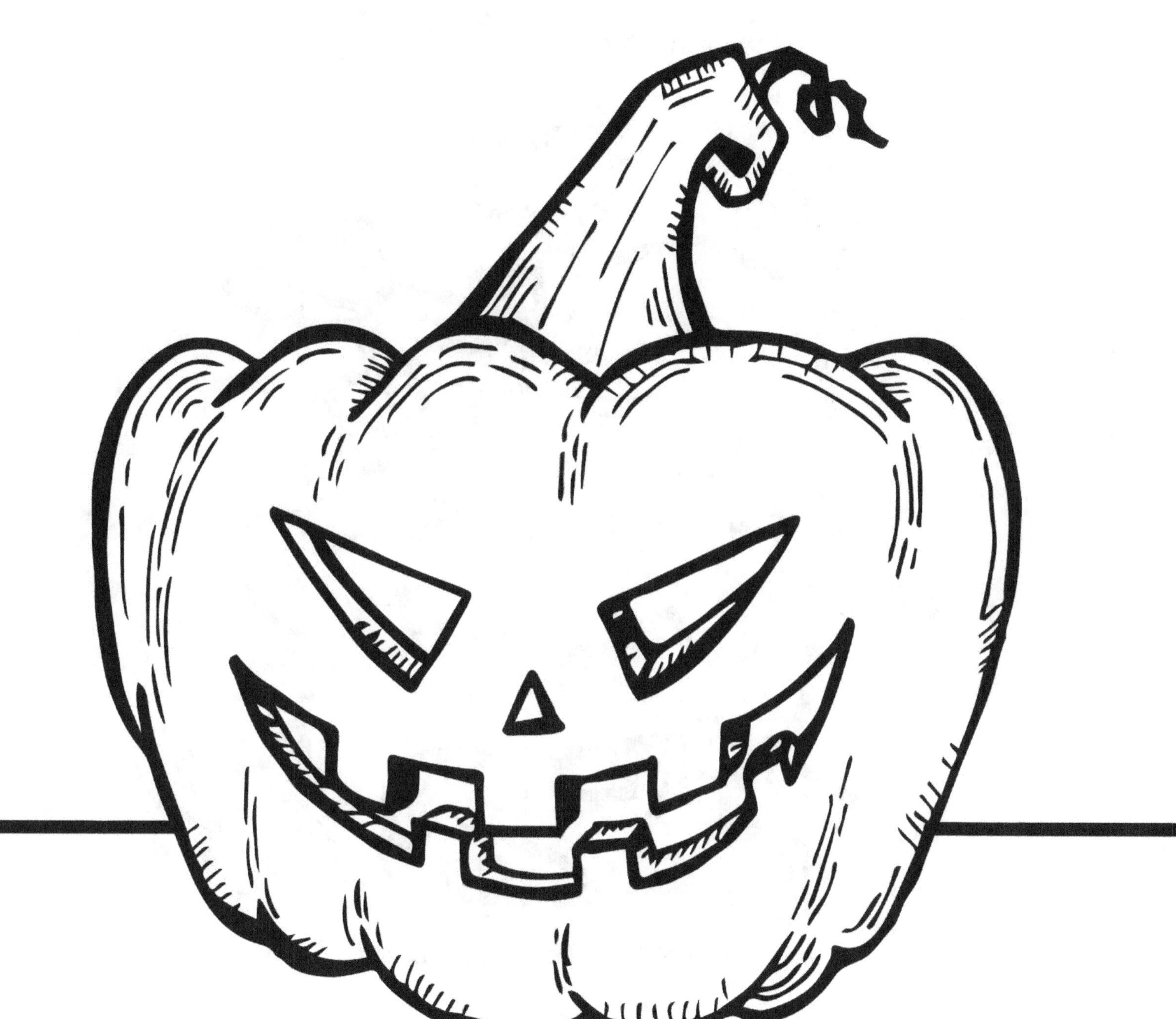

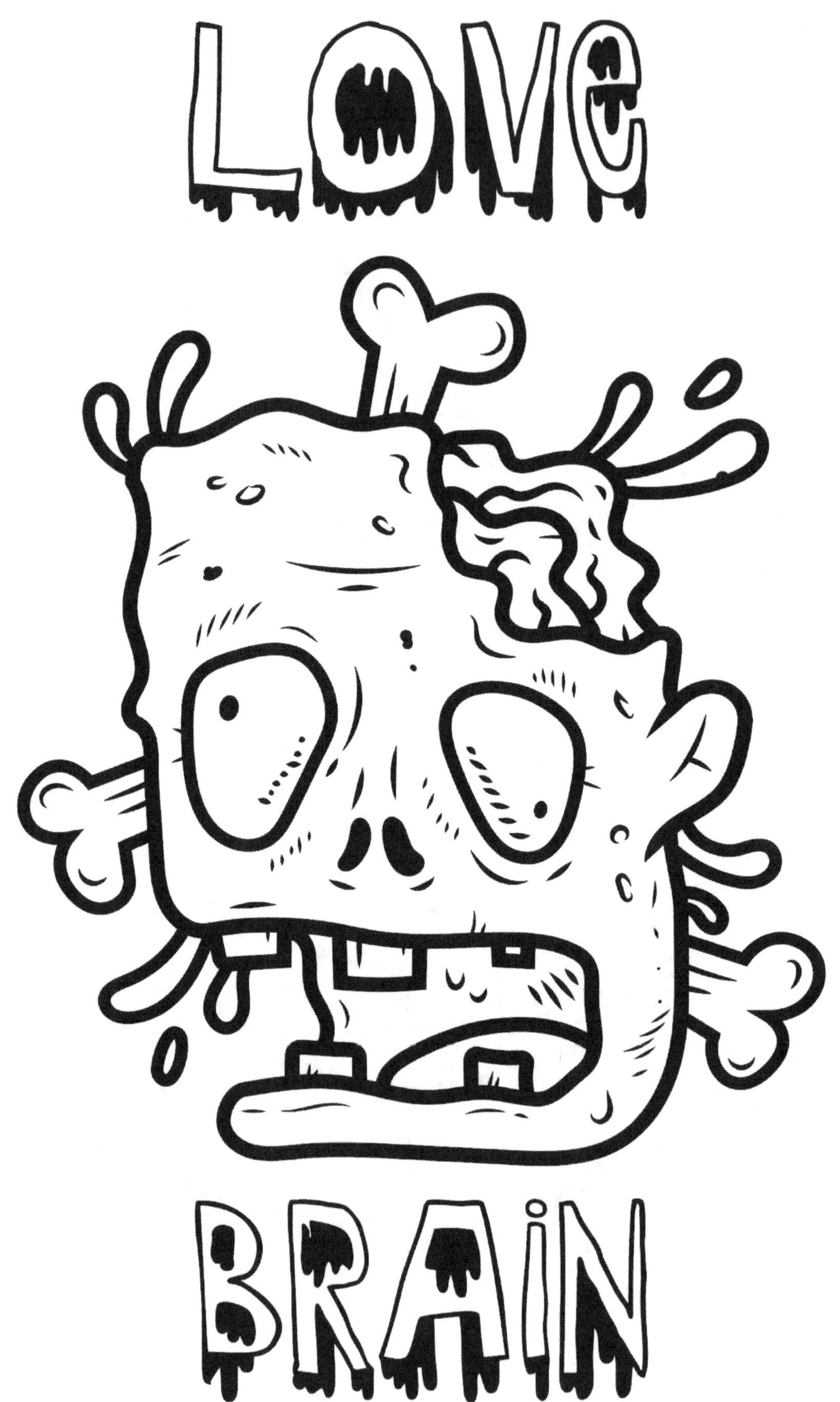

LOVE
BRAIN

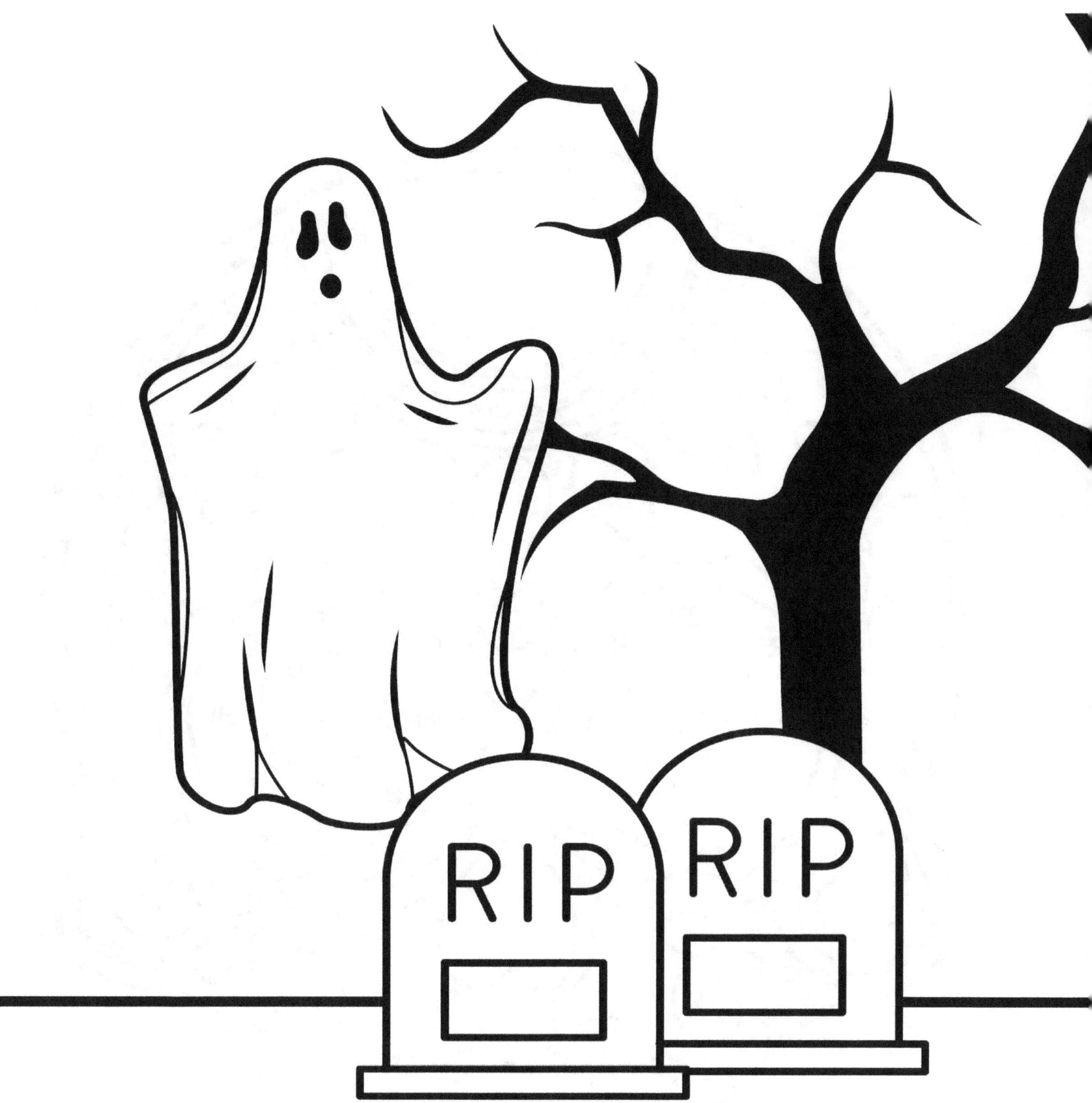
RIP
RIP

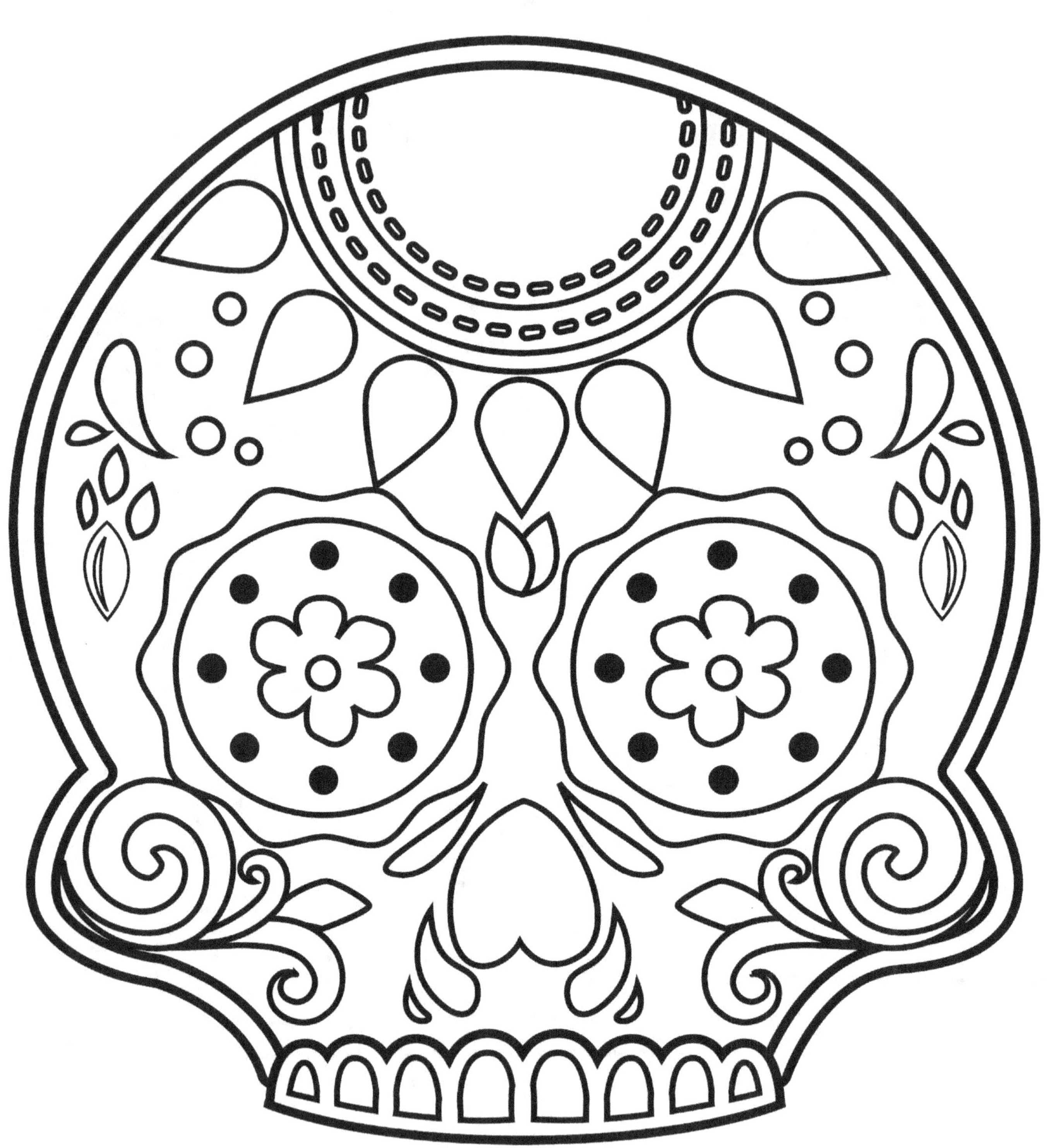

Happy Halloween

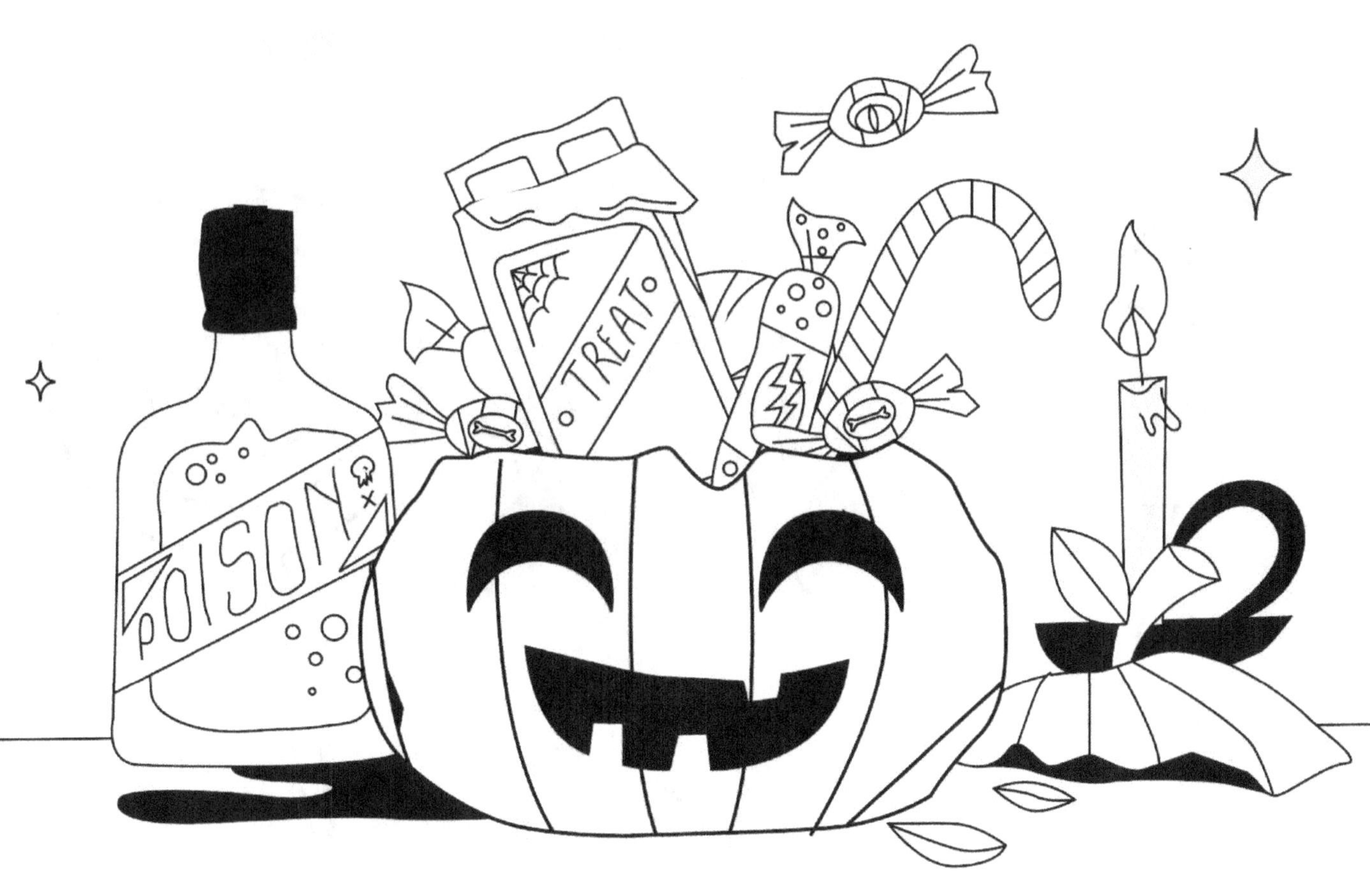

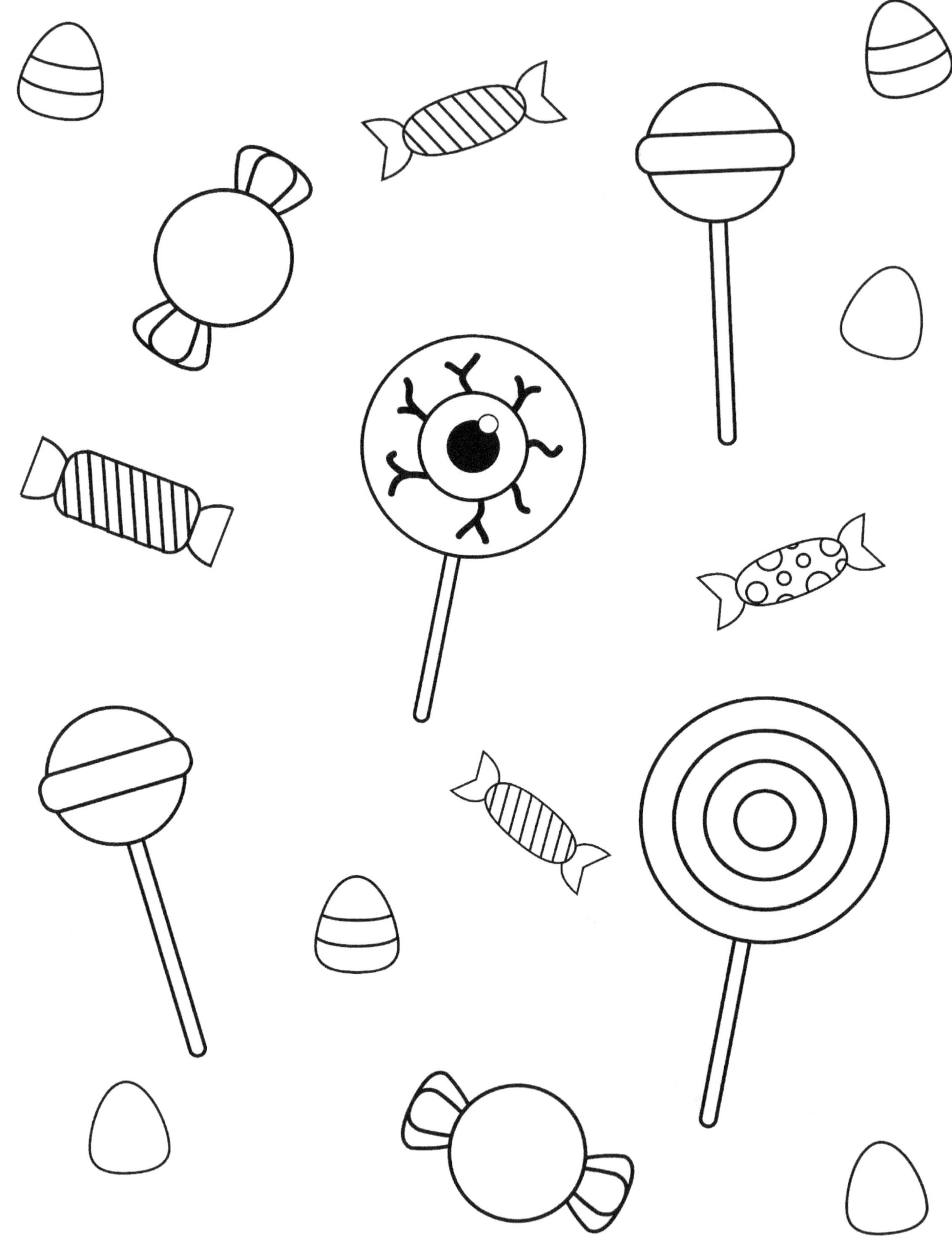

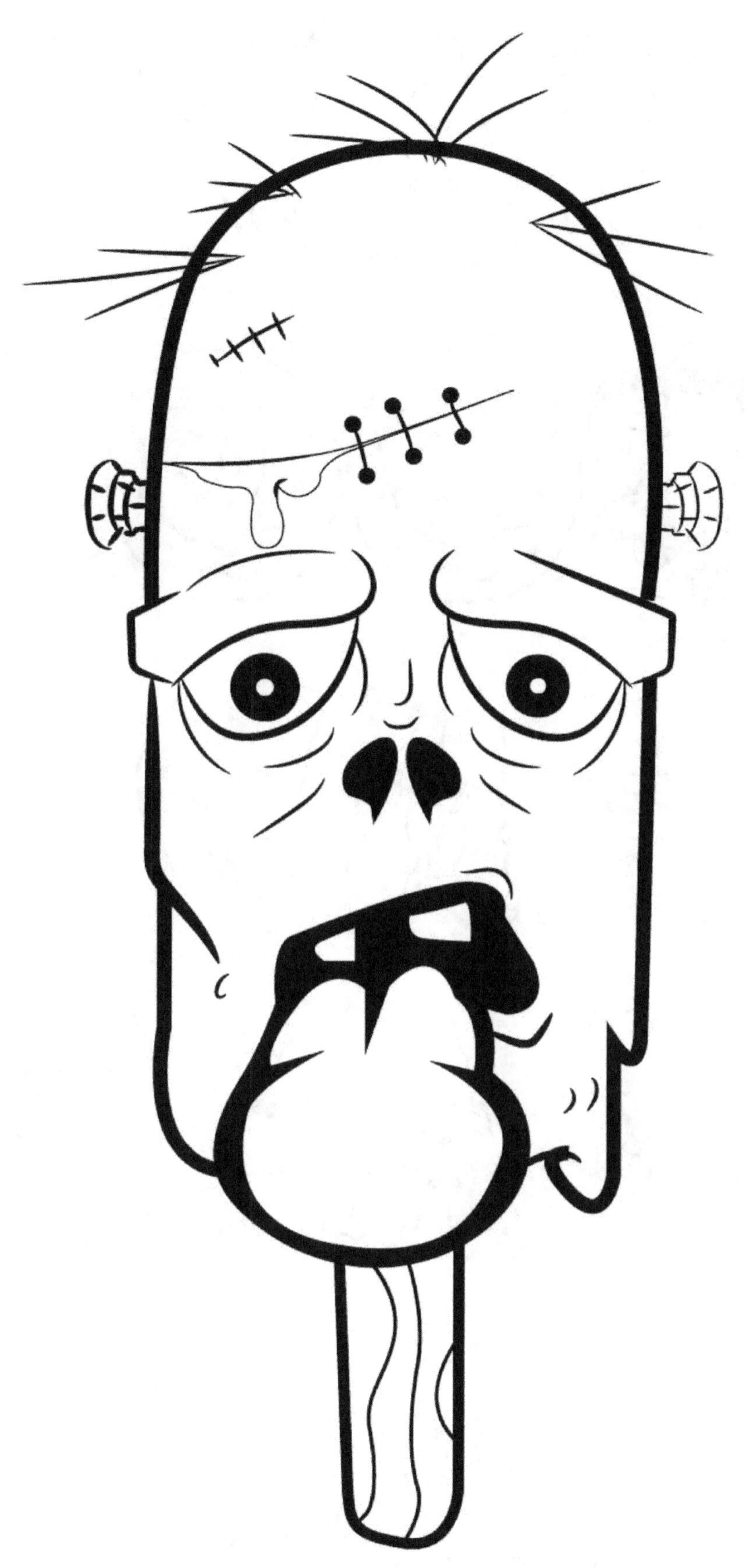

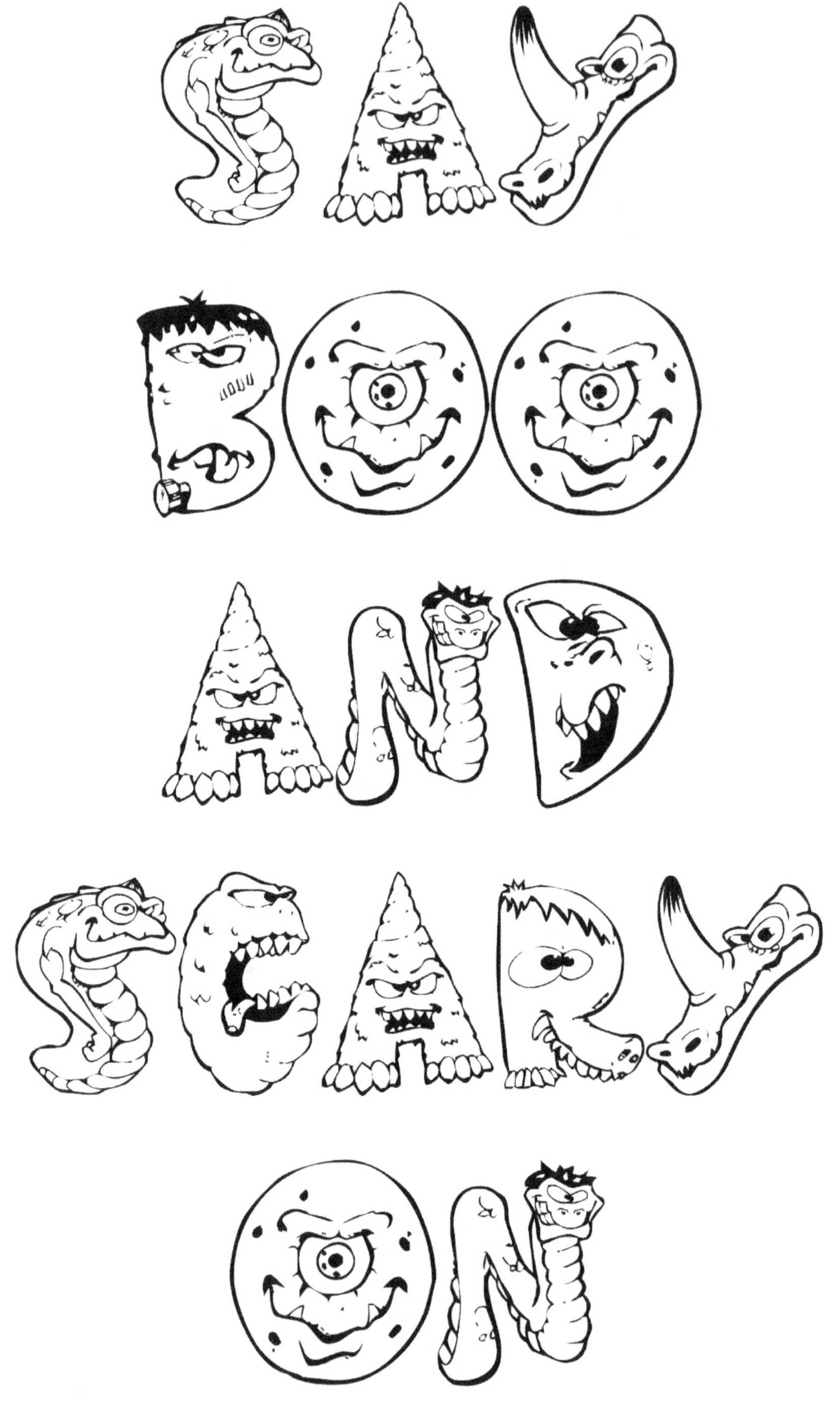

SAY
BOO
AND
SCARY
ON

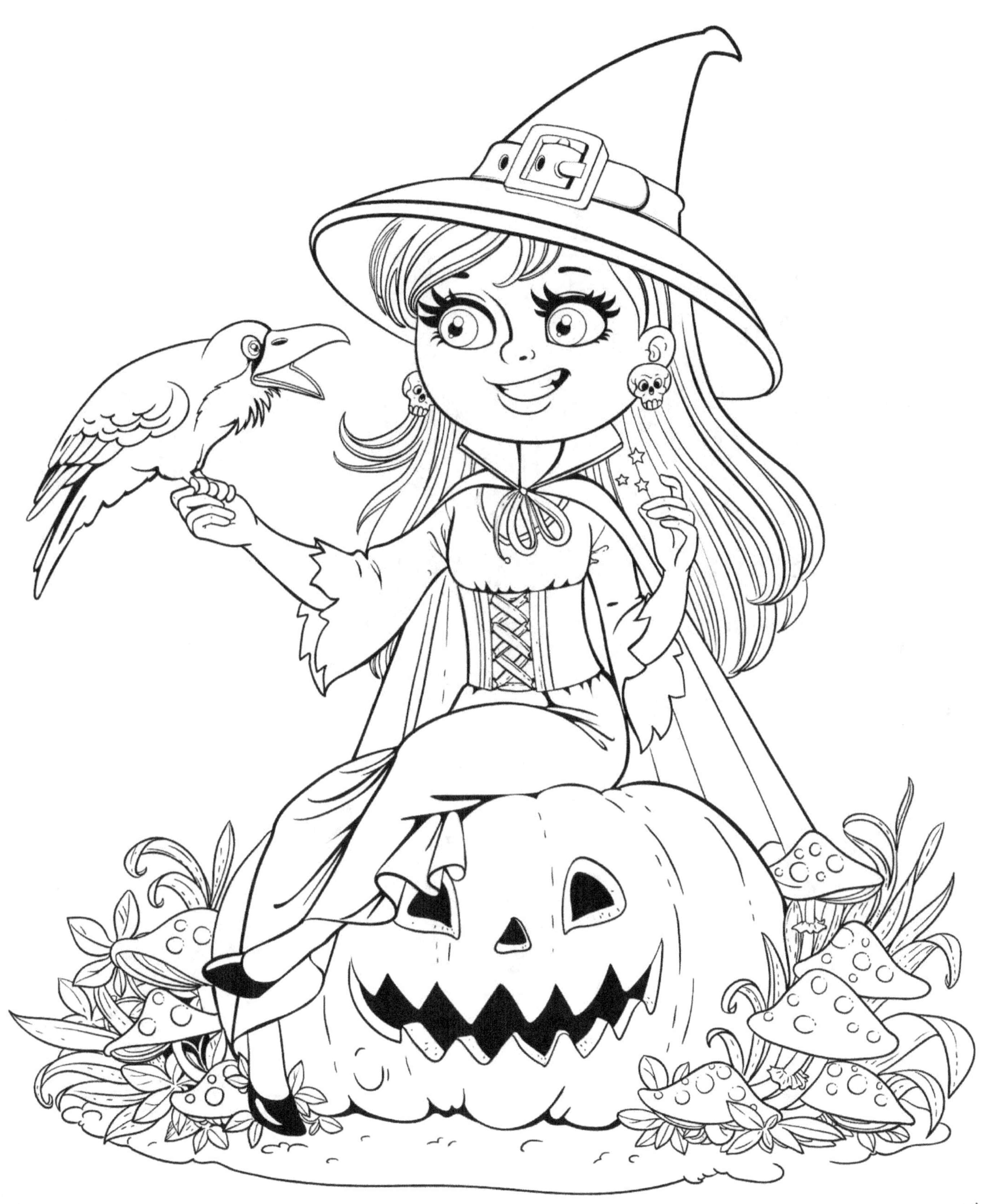

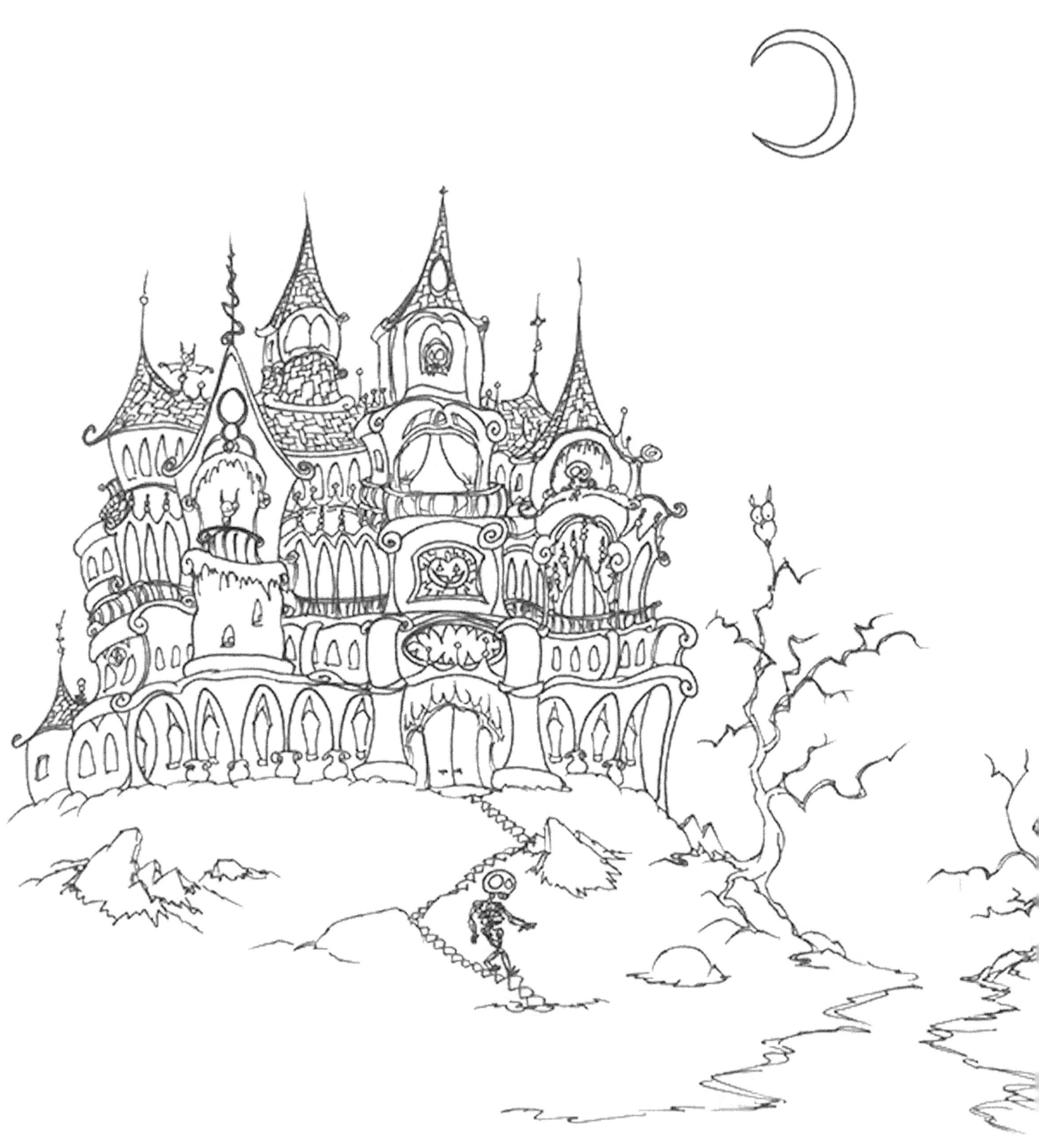

CONNECT THE DOTS TO FINISH THE PICTURE!

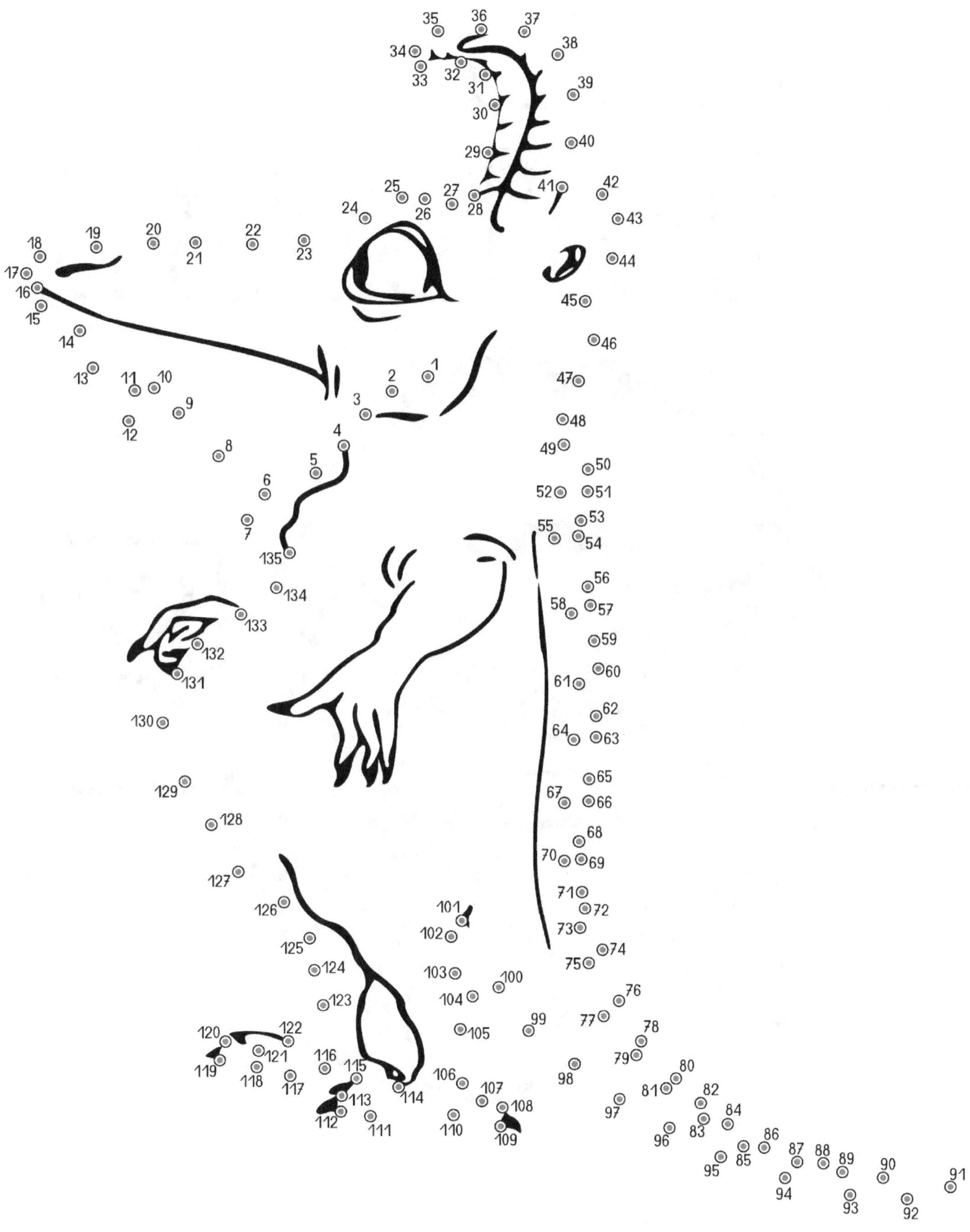

LITTLE MONSTER

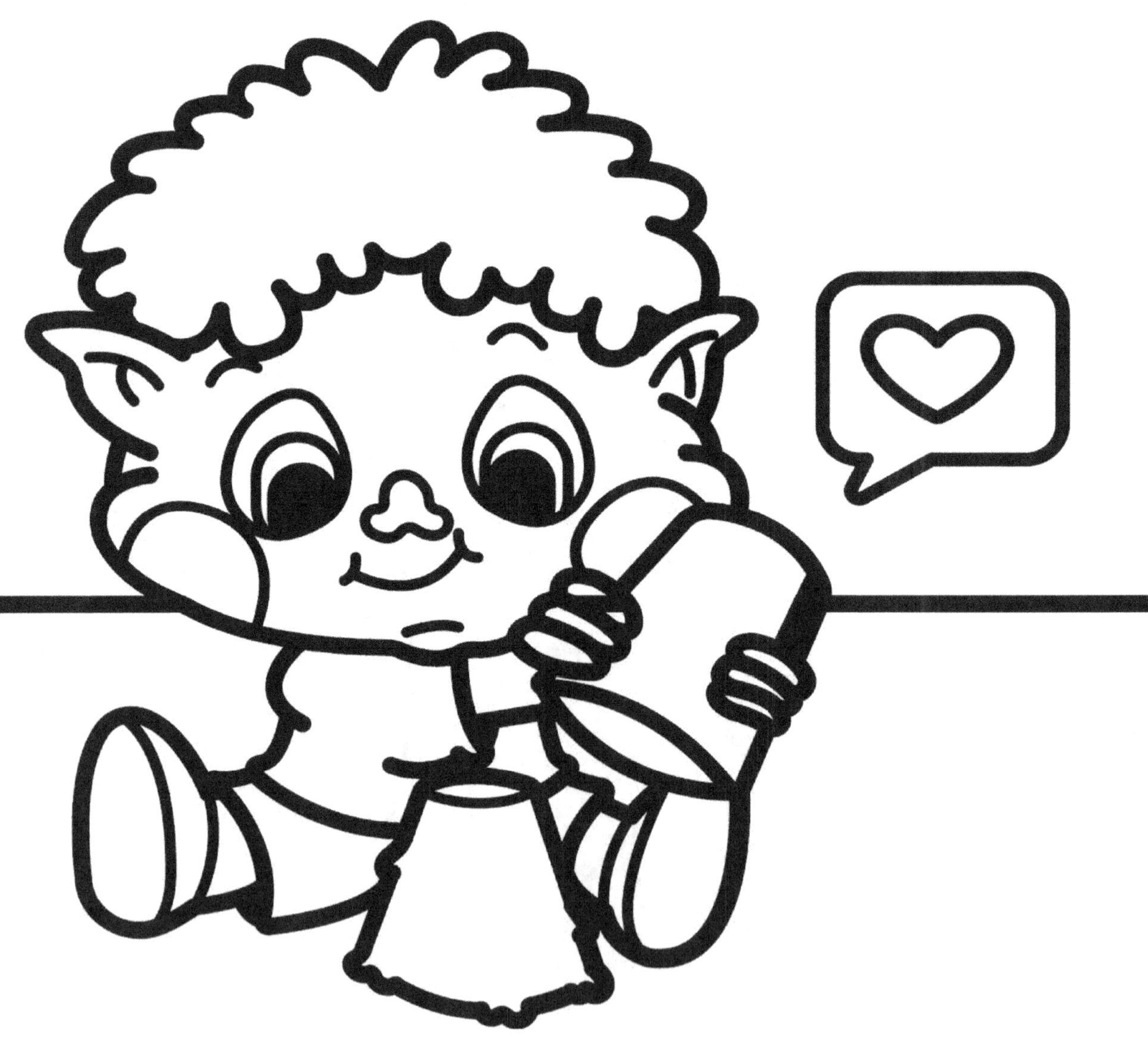

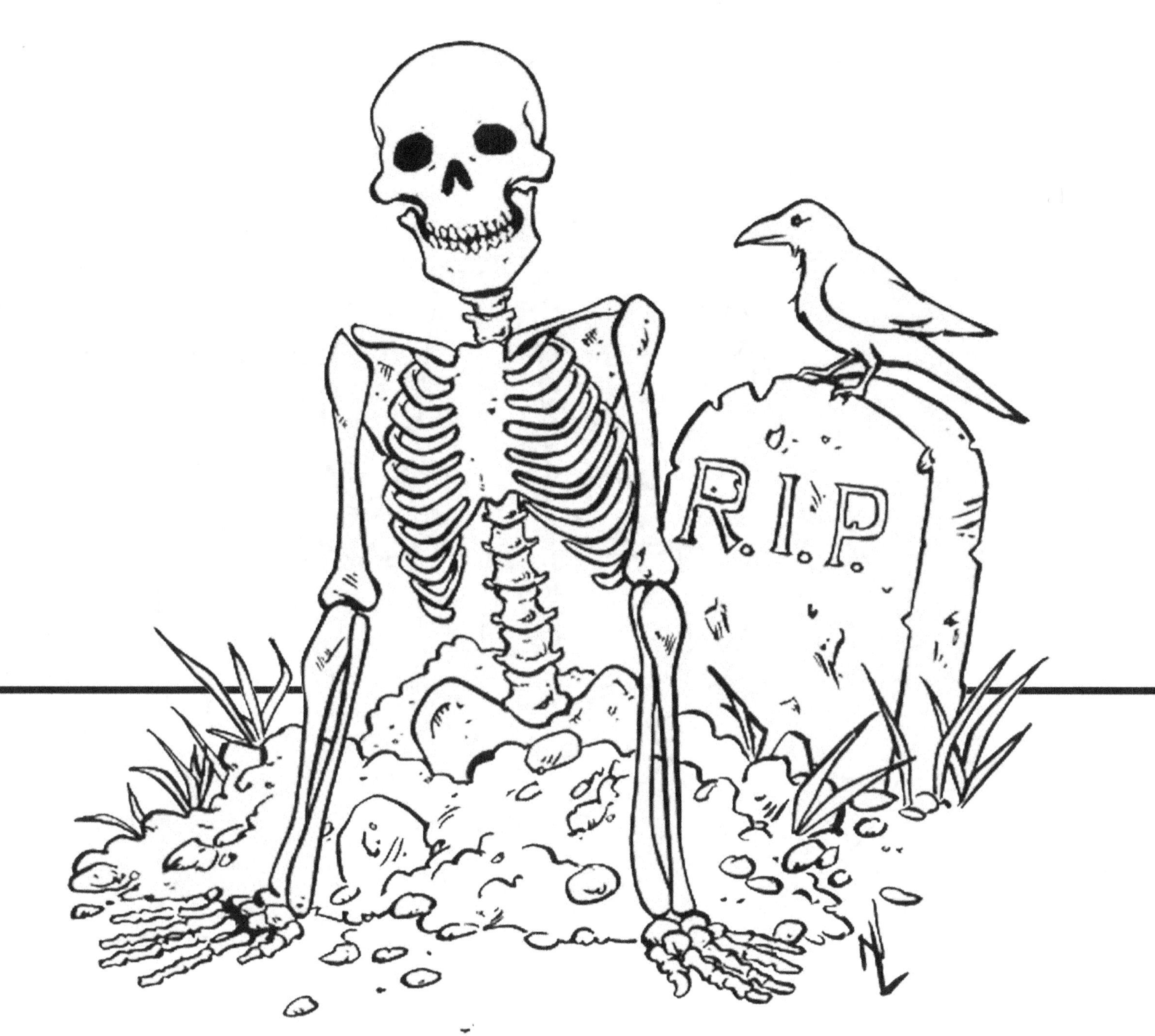
R.I.P

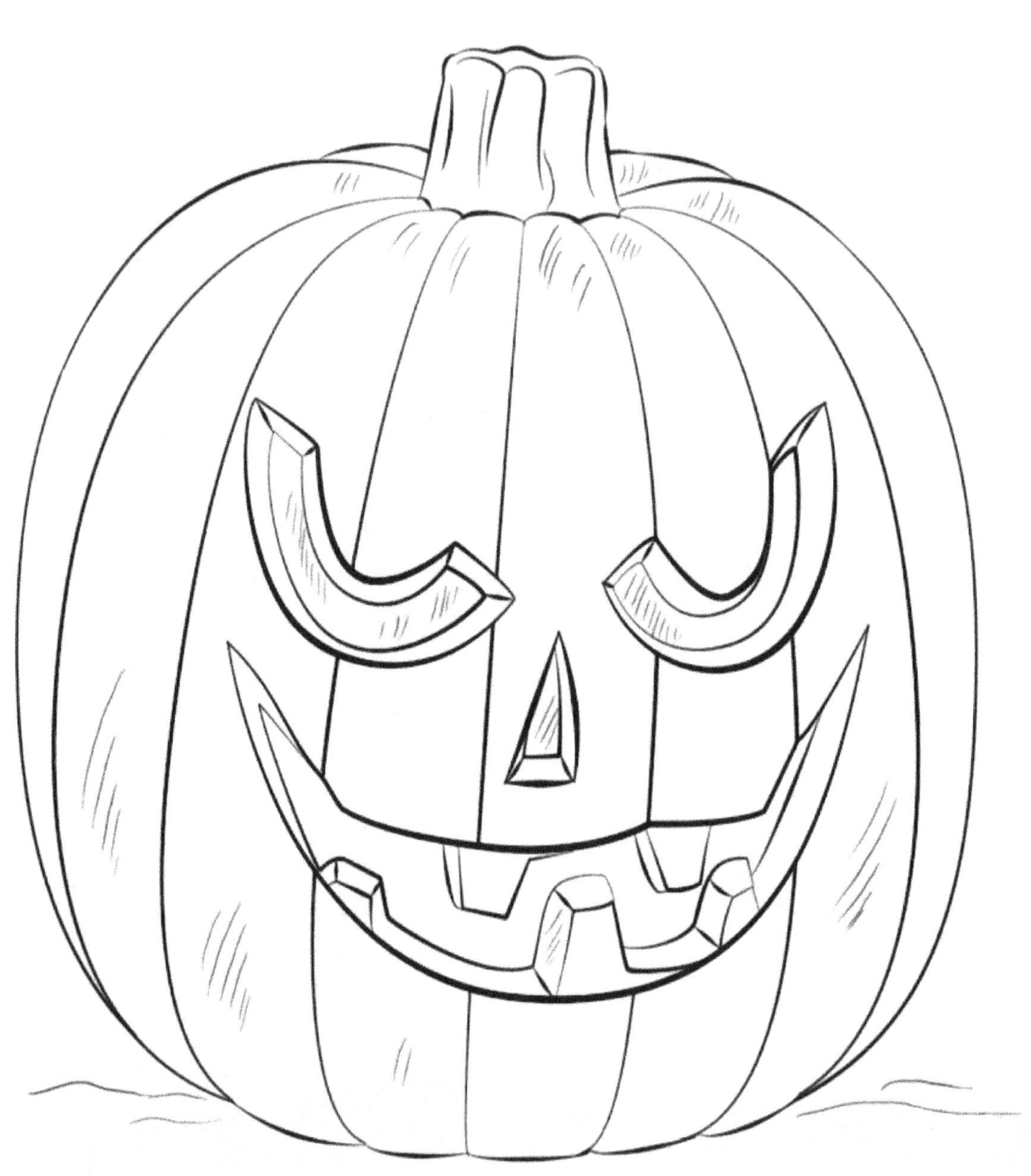

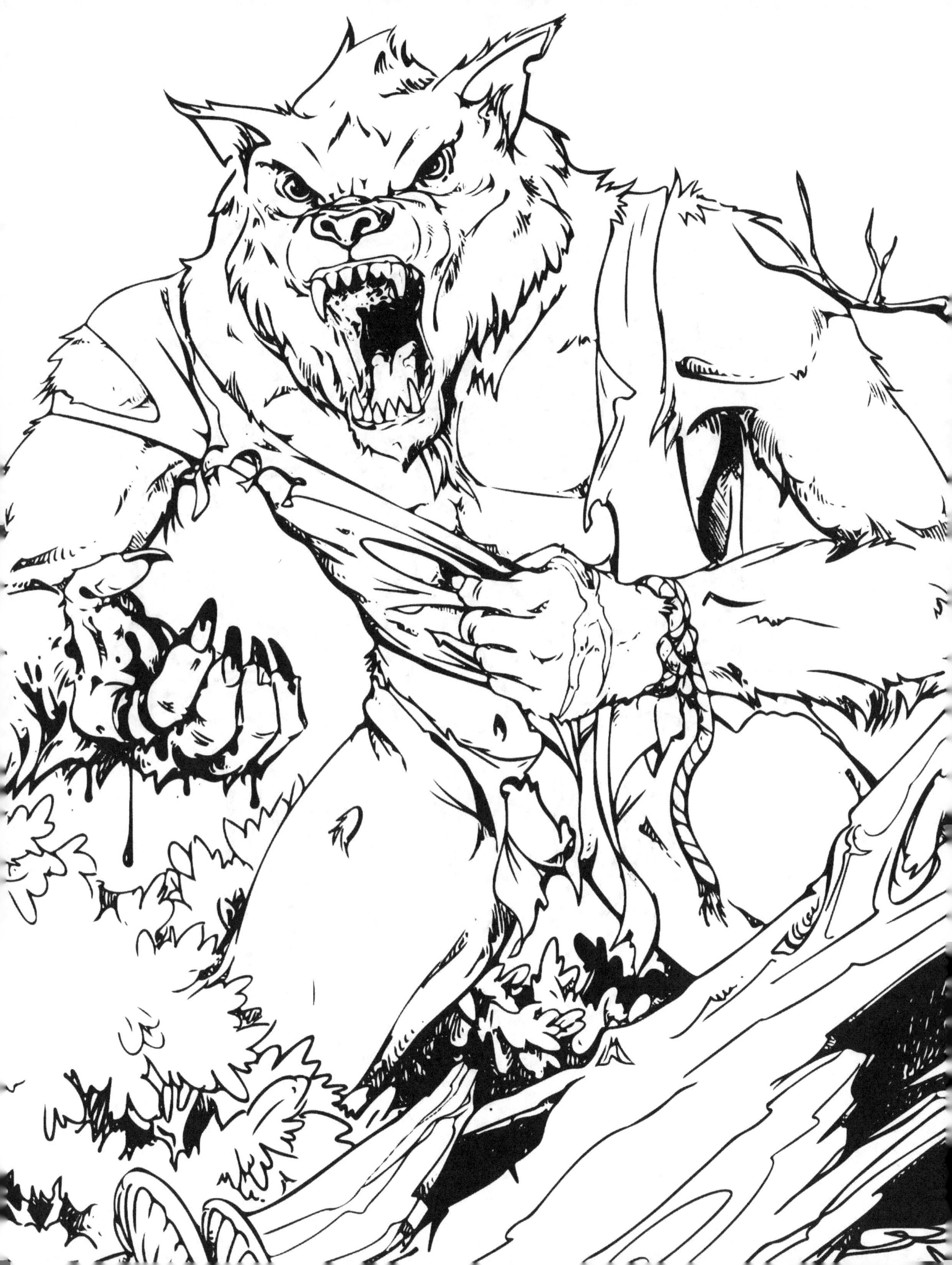

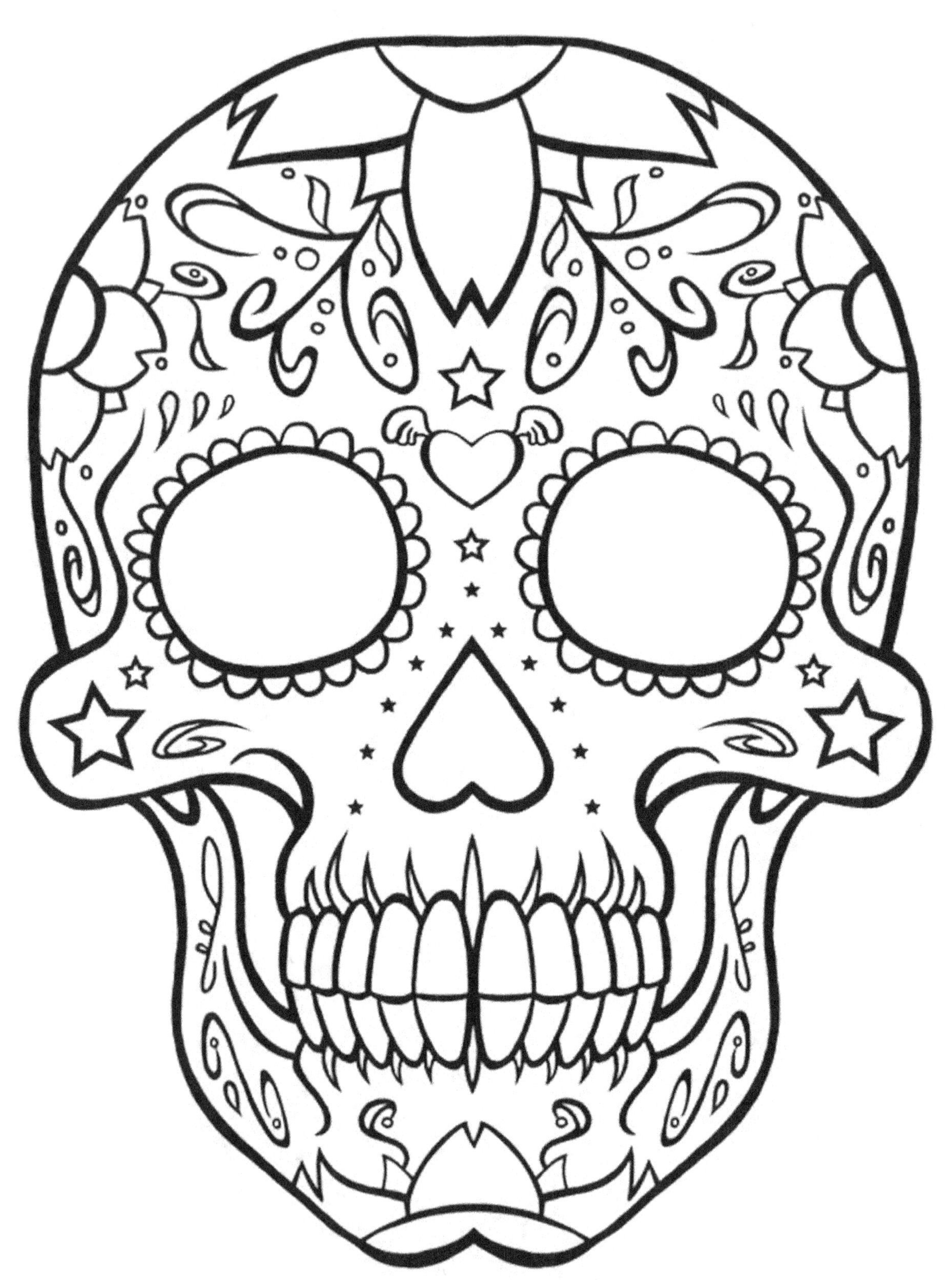

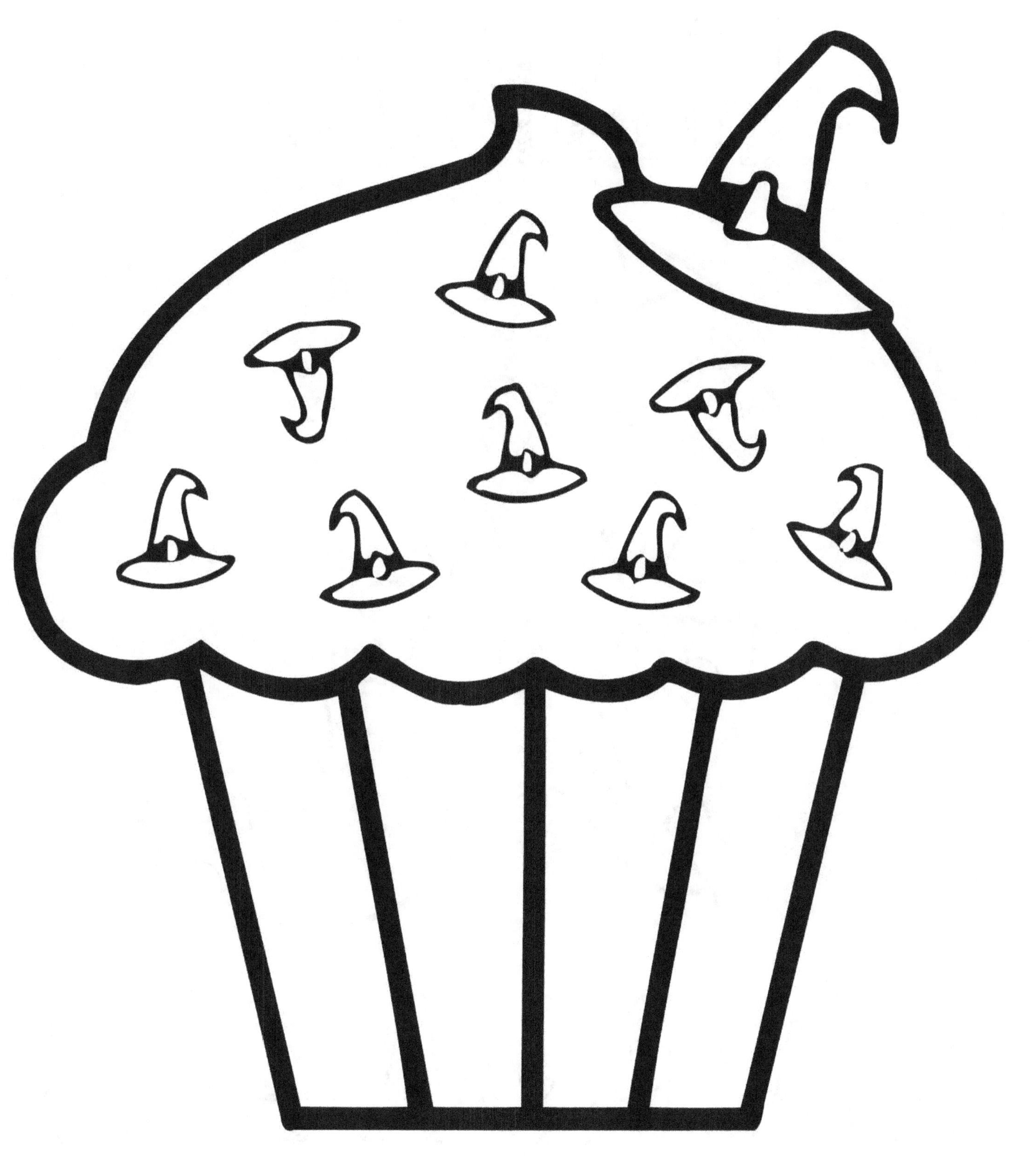

HAPPY

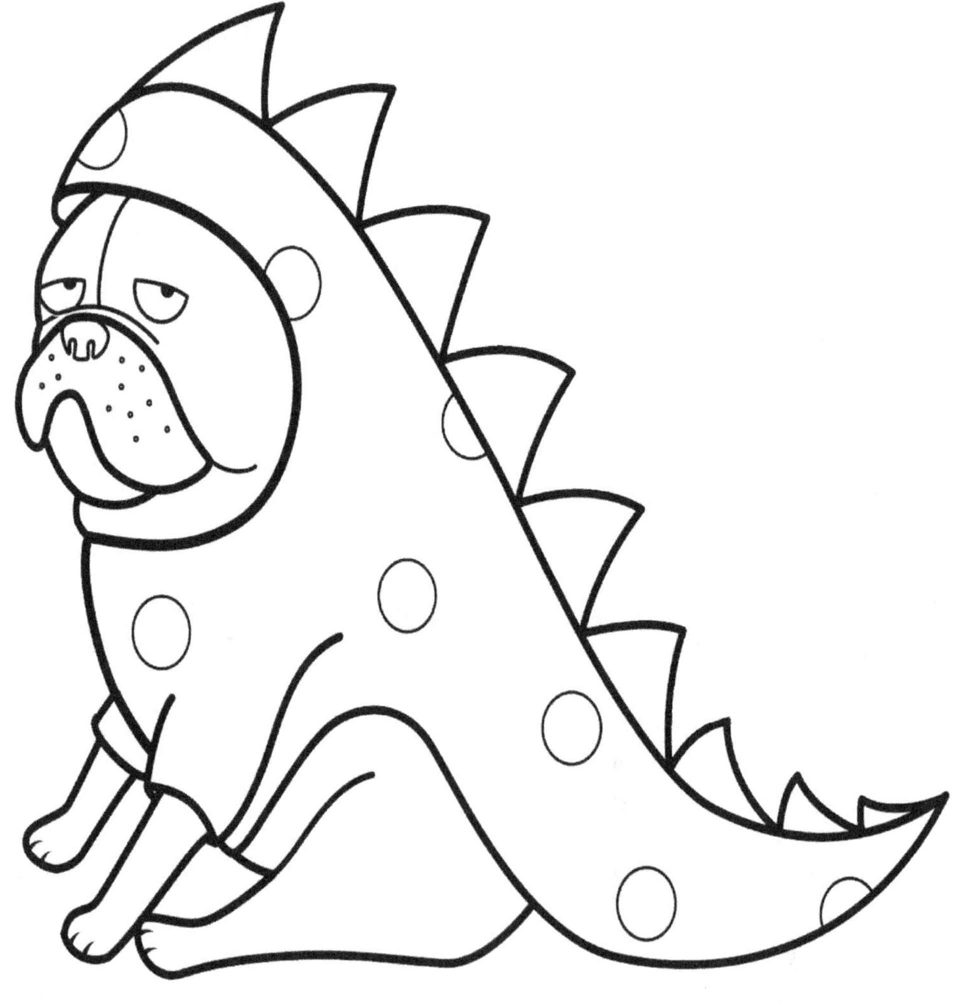

HALLOWEEN

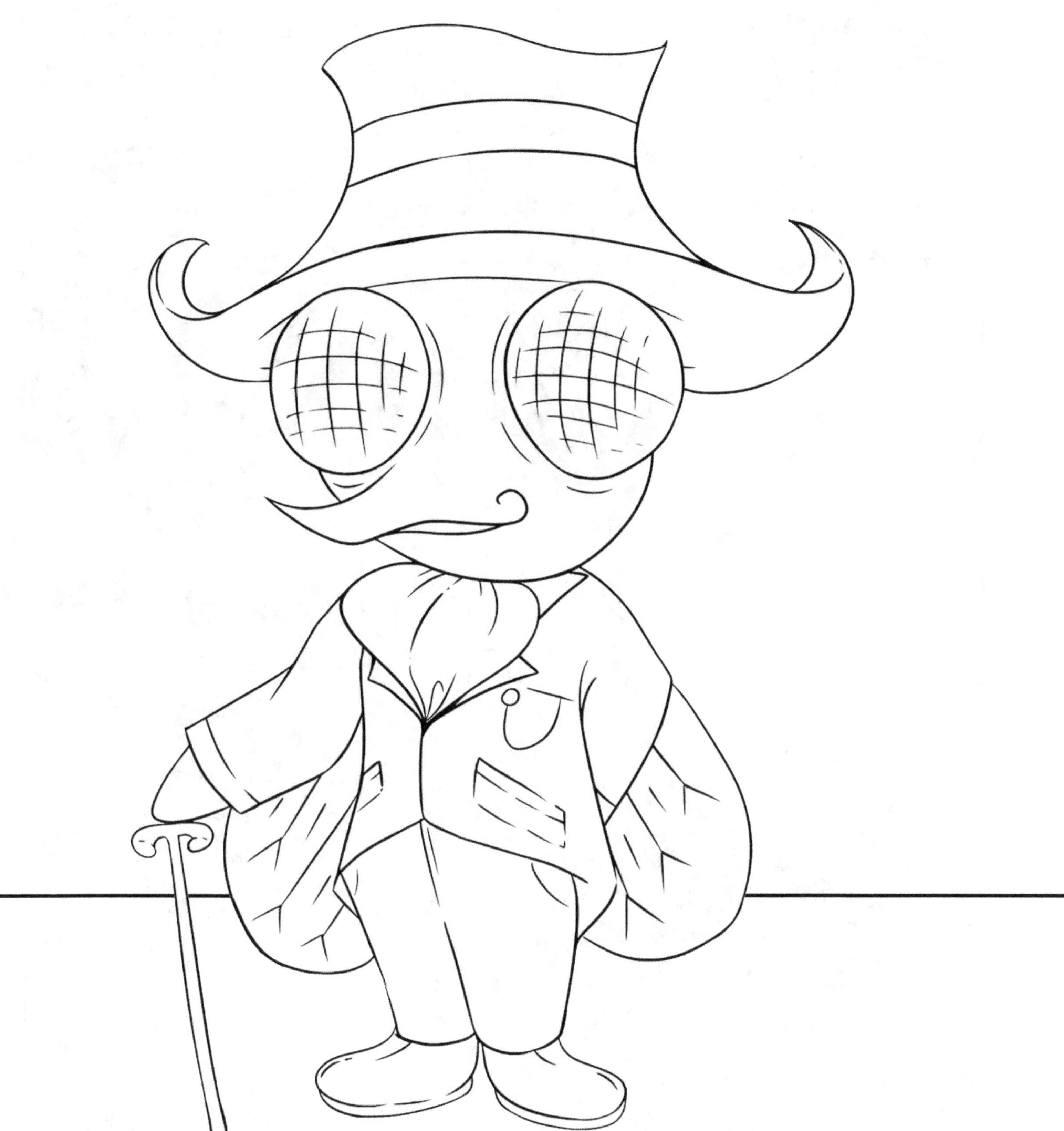

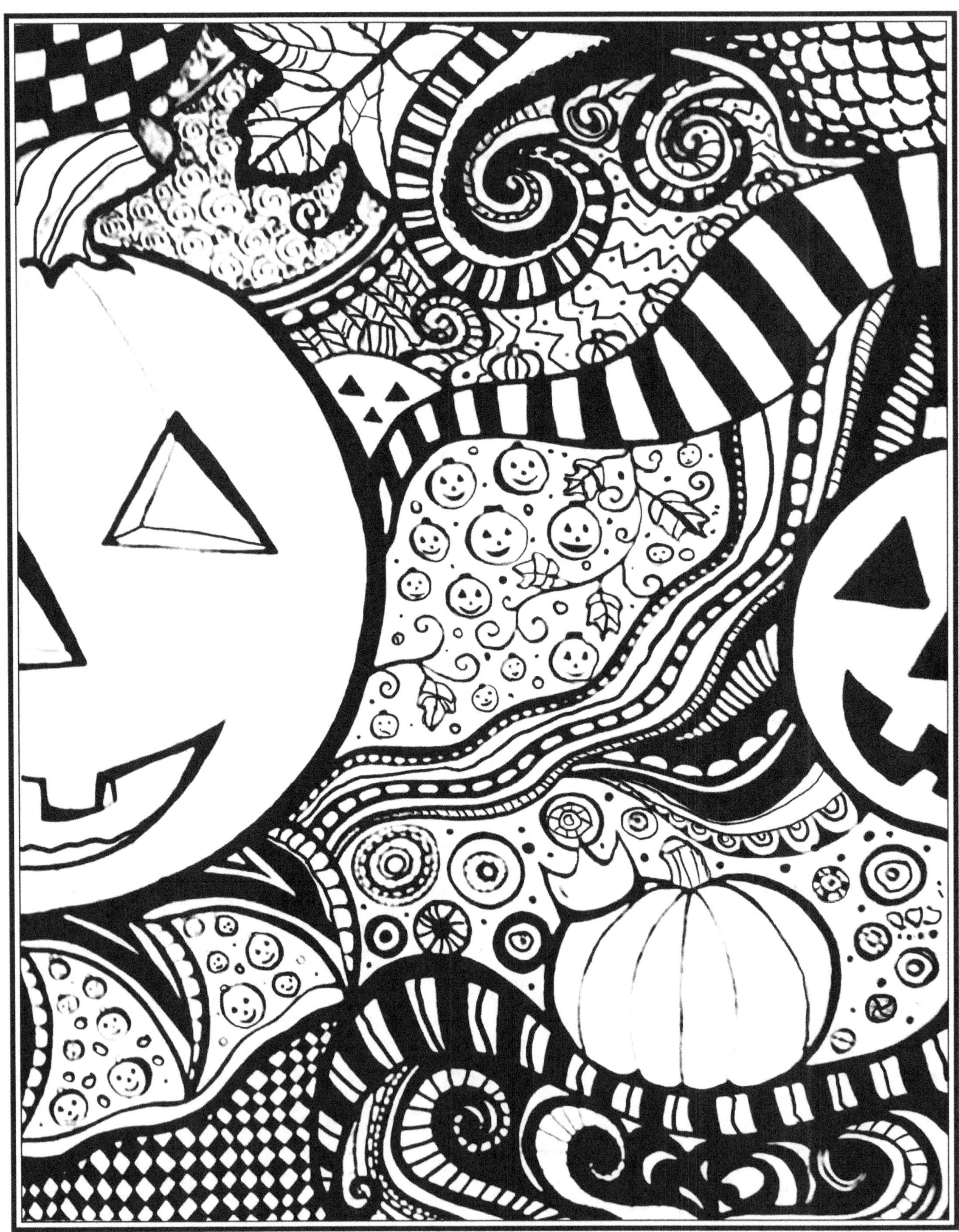

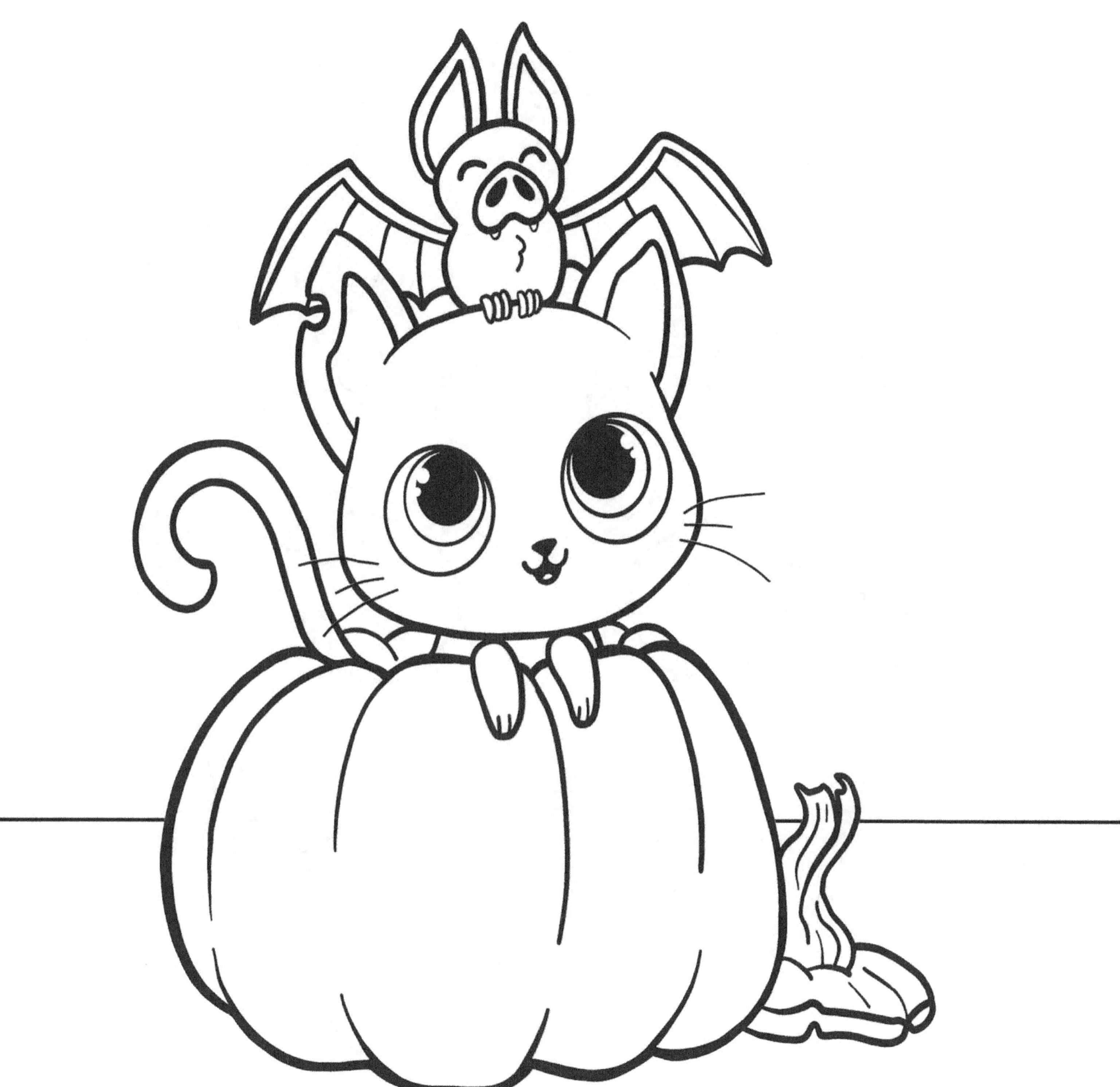

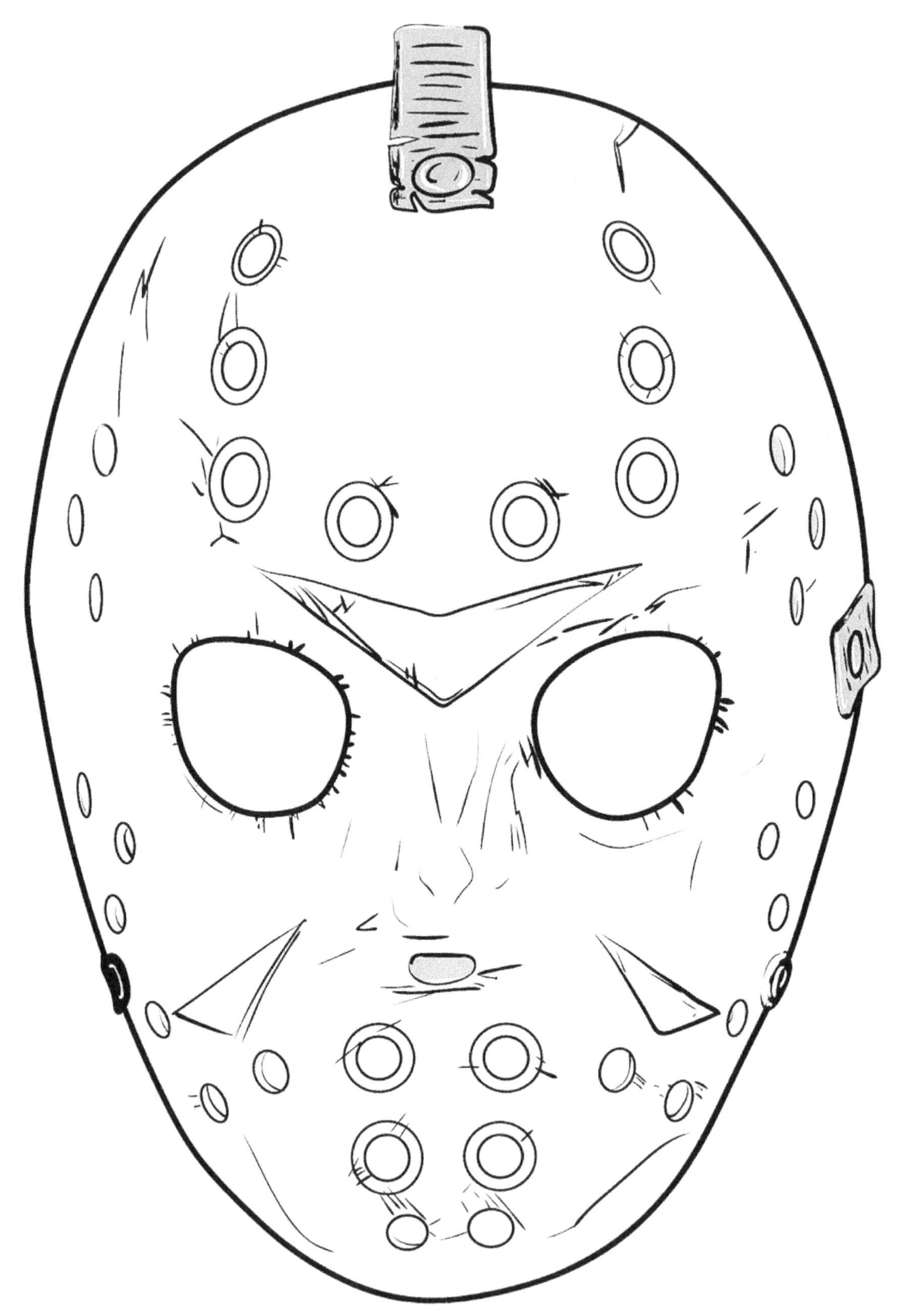

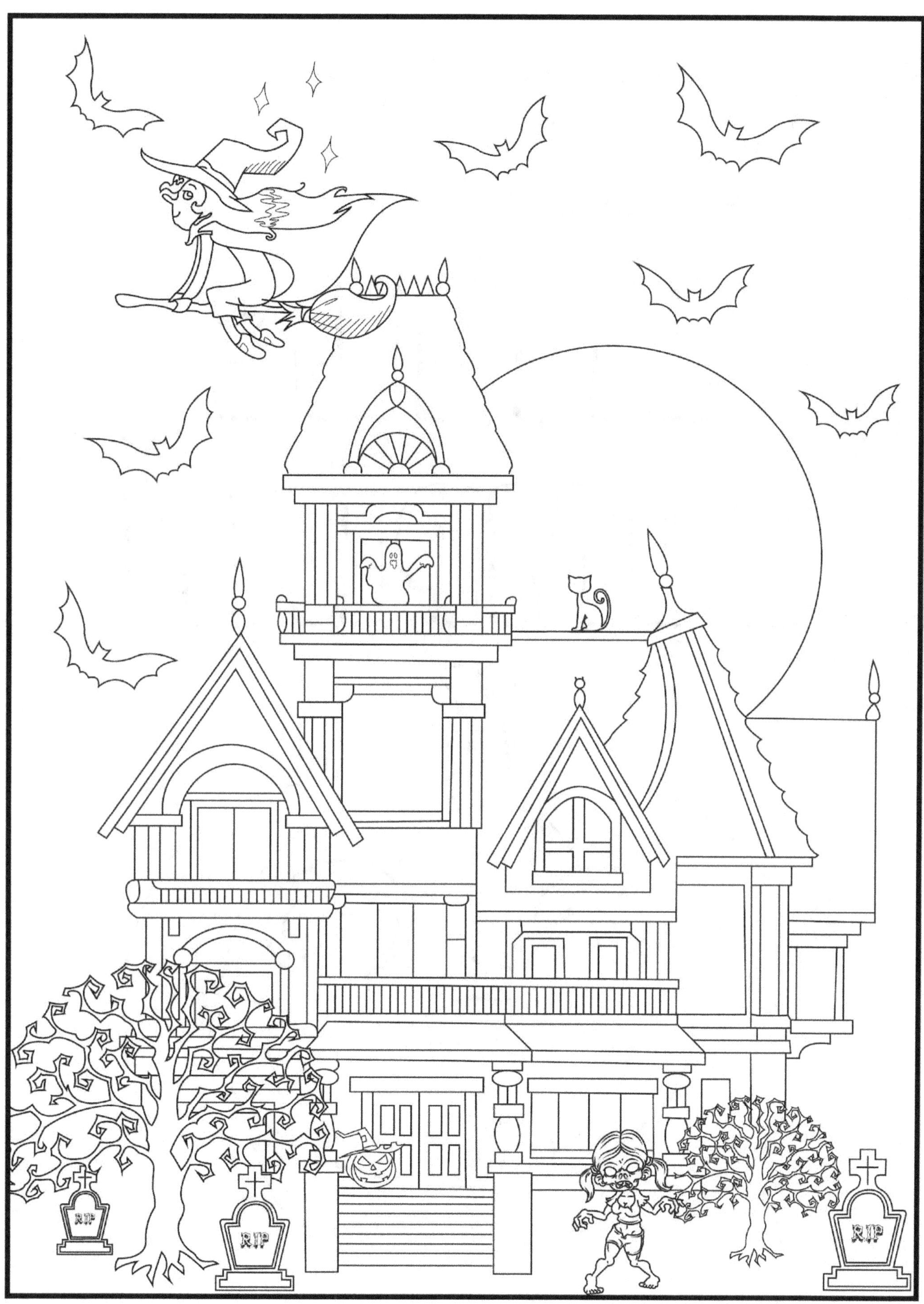

DADDY'S LITTLE PUMPKIN

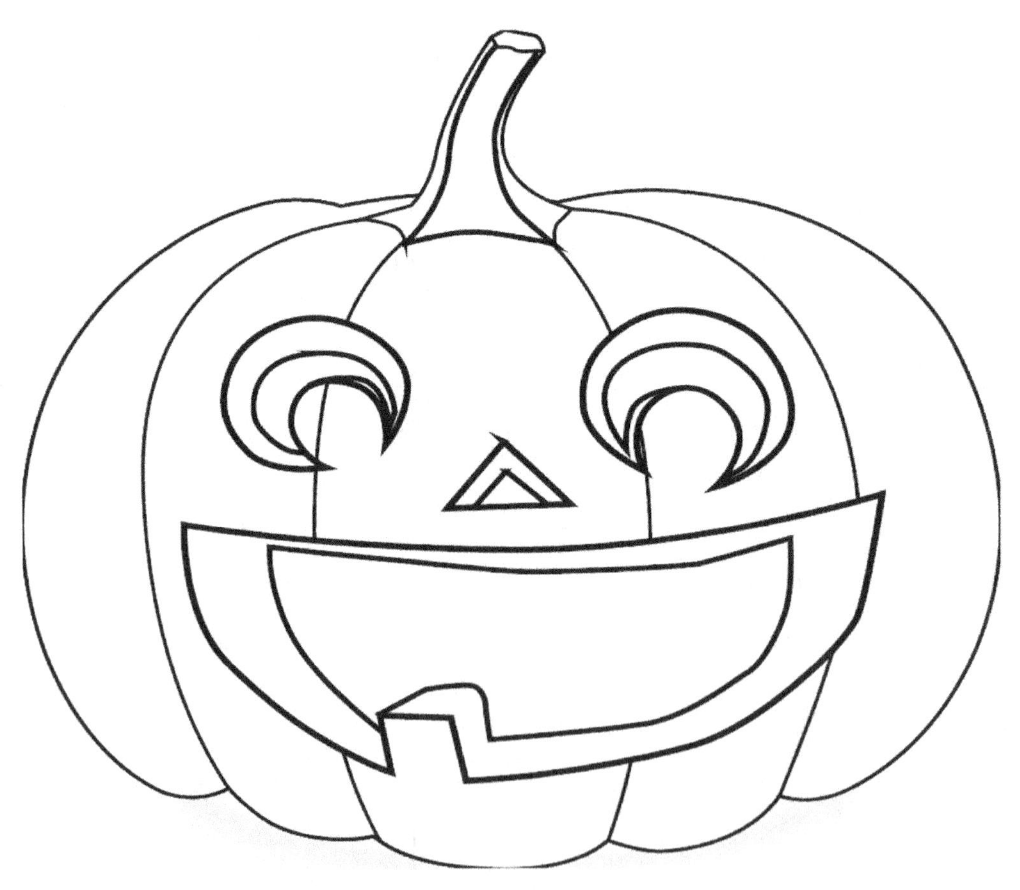

LITTLE
ZOMBIE

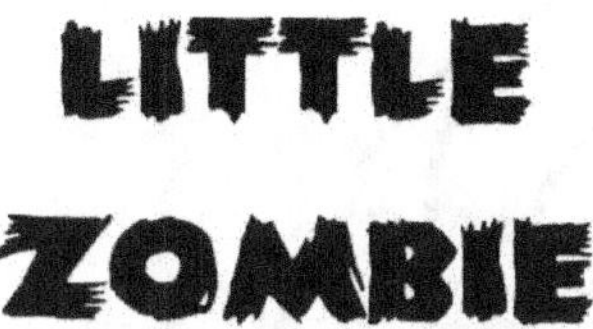
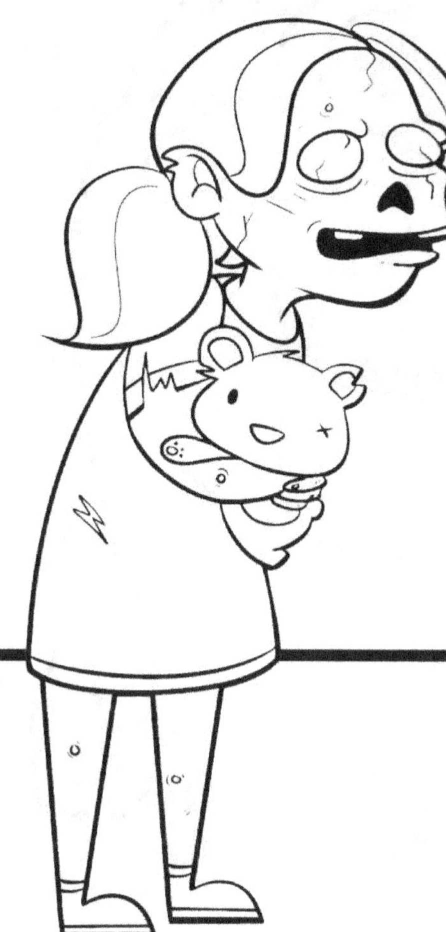

DADDY
ZOMBIE

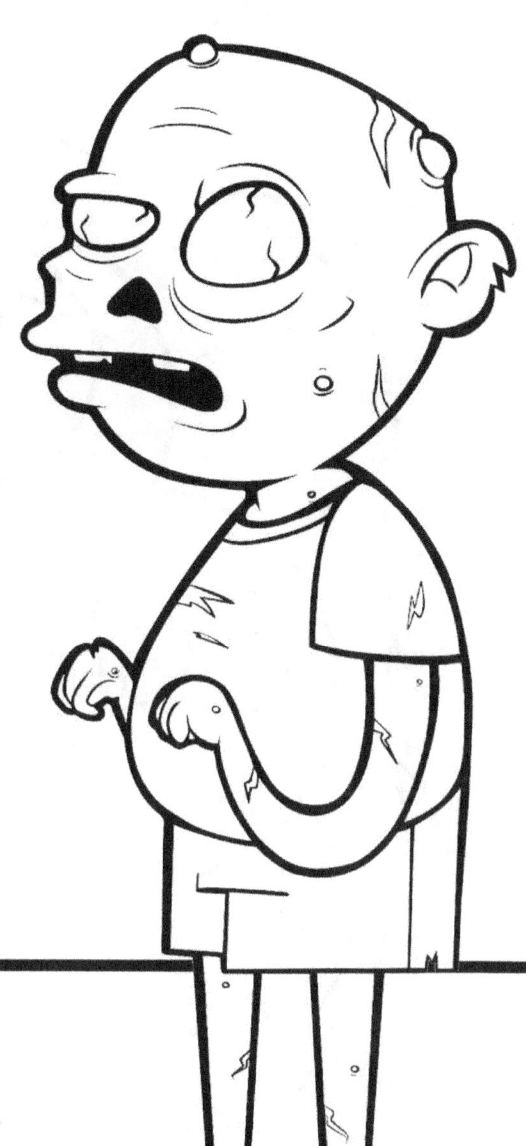

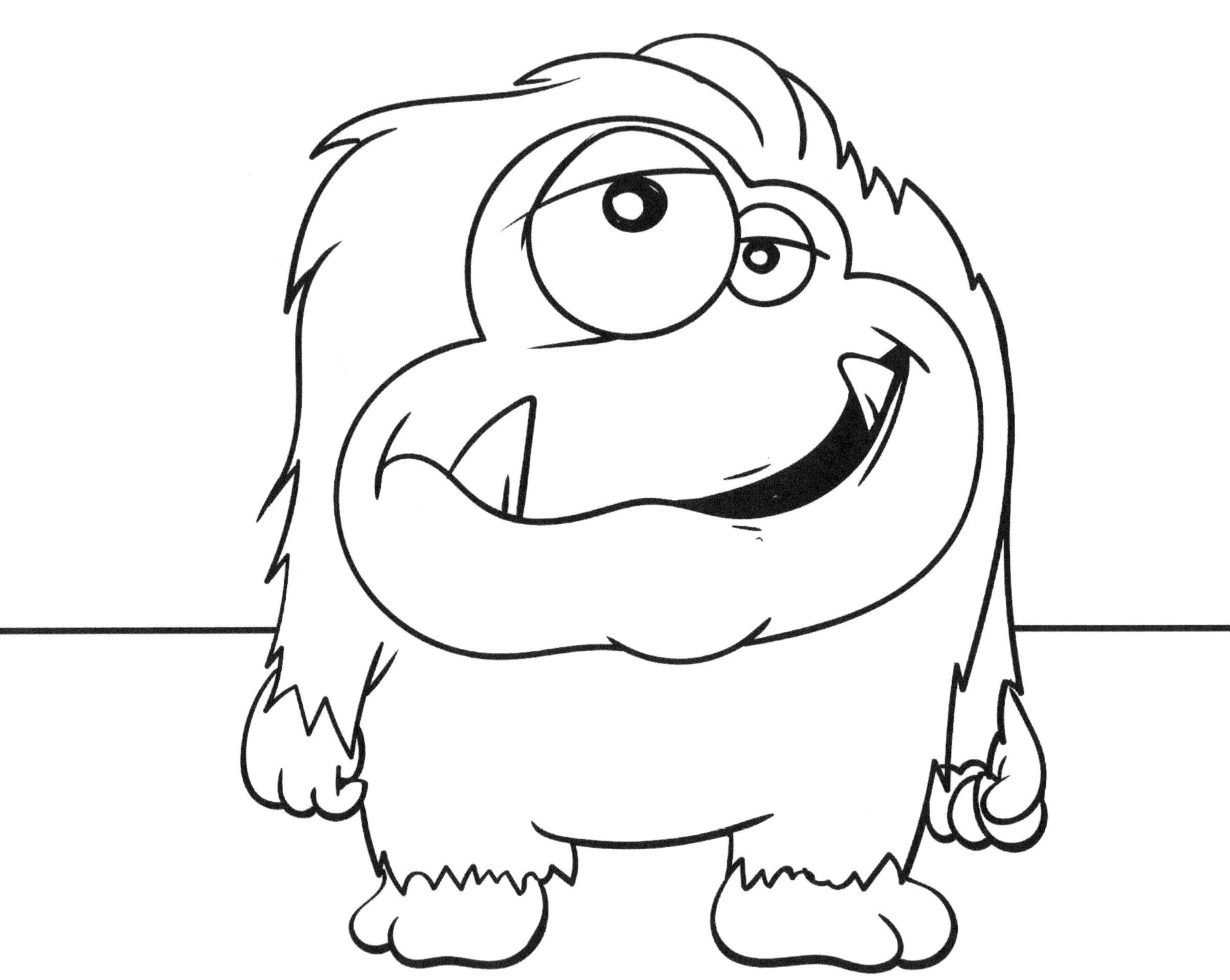

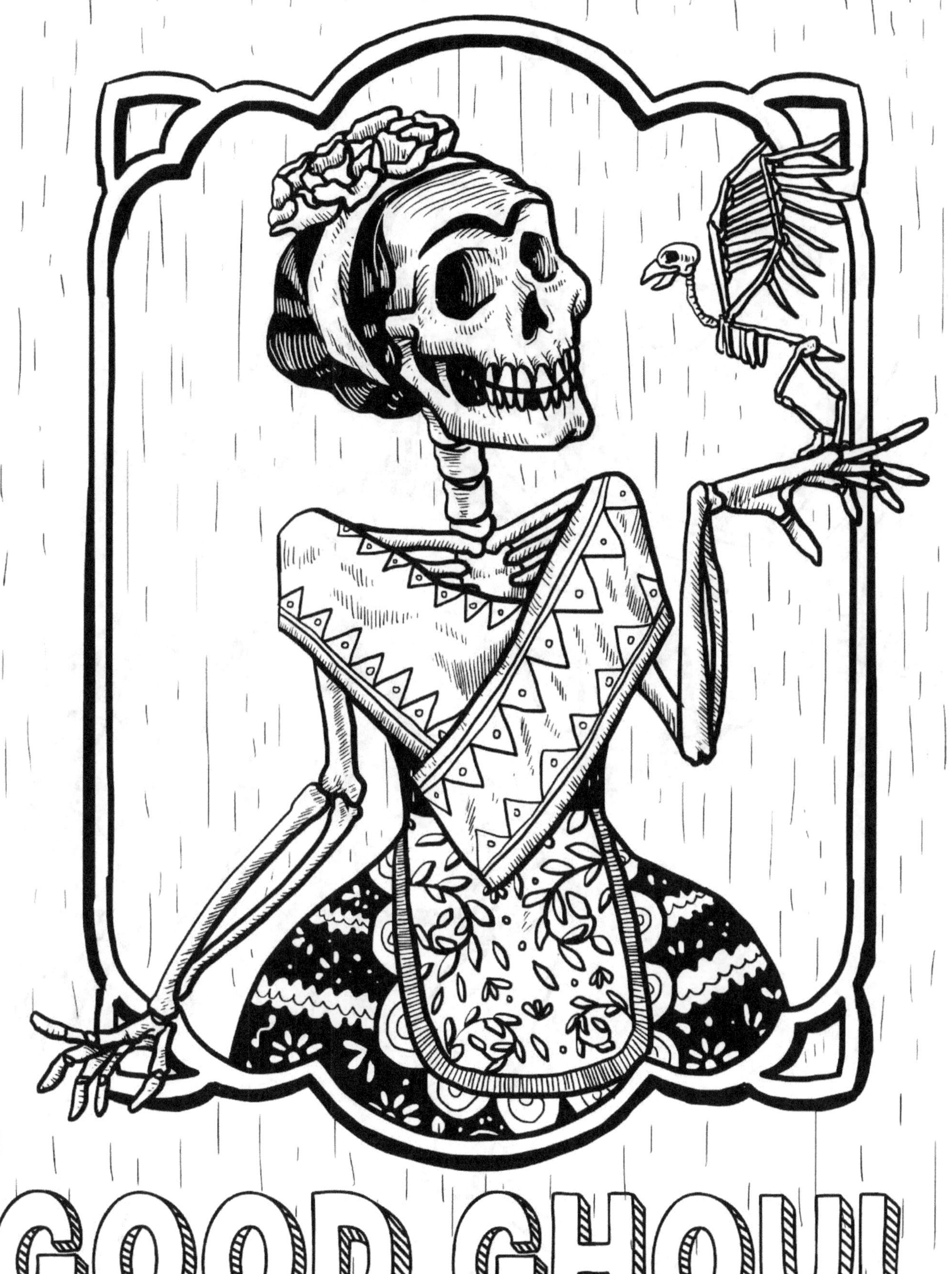

GOOD GHOUL

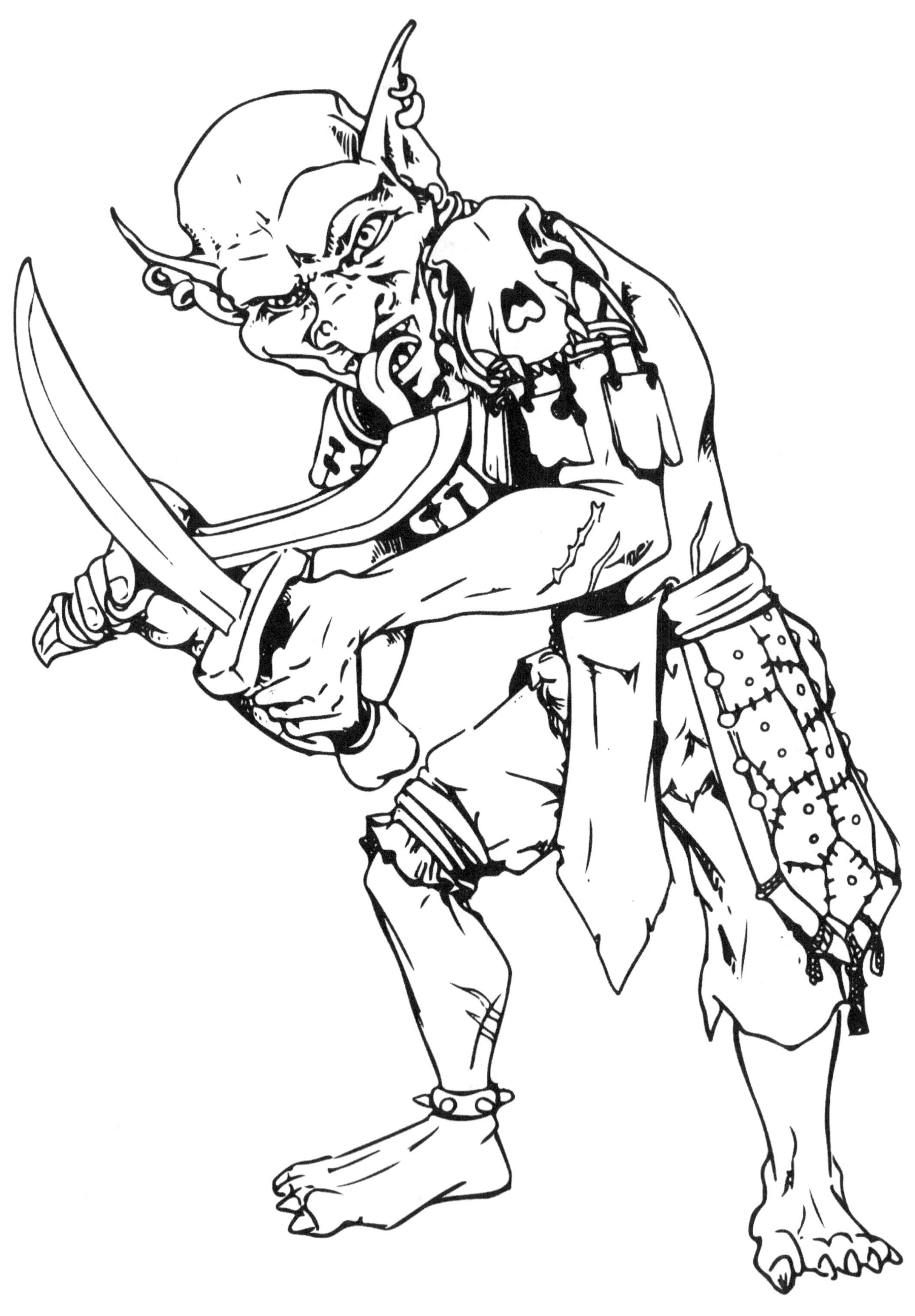

WITCHY KITTY

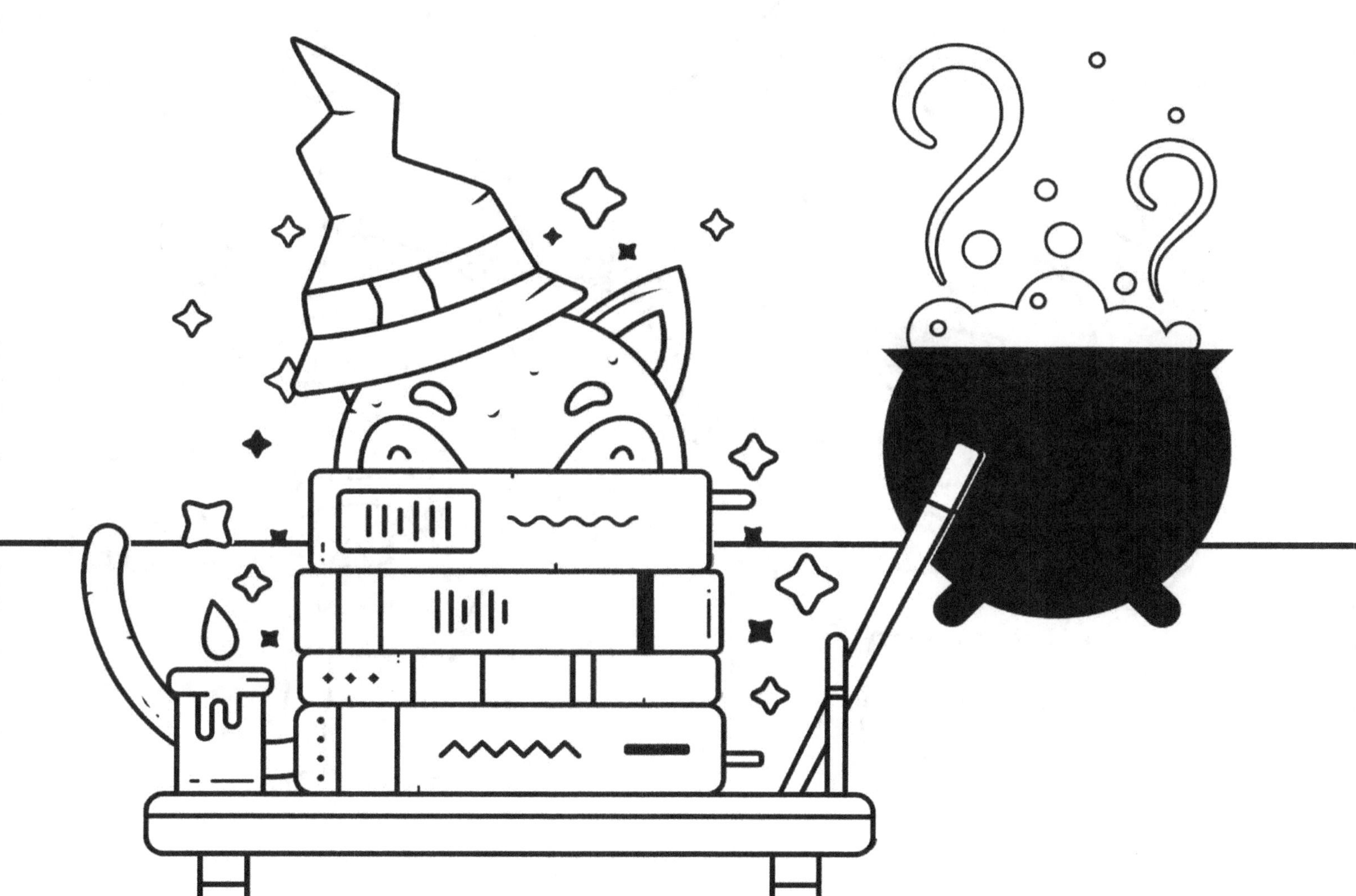

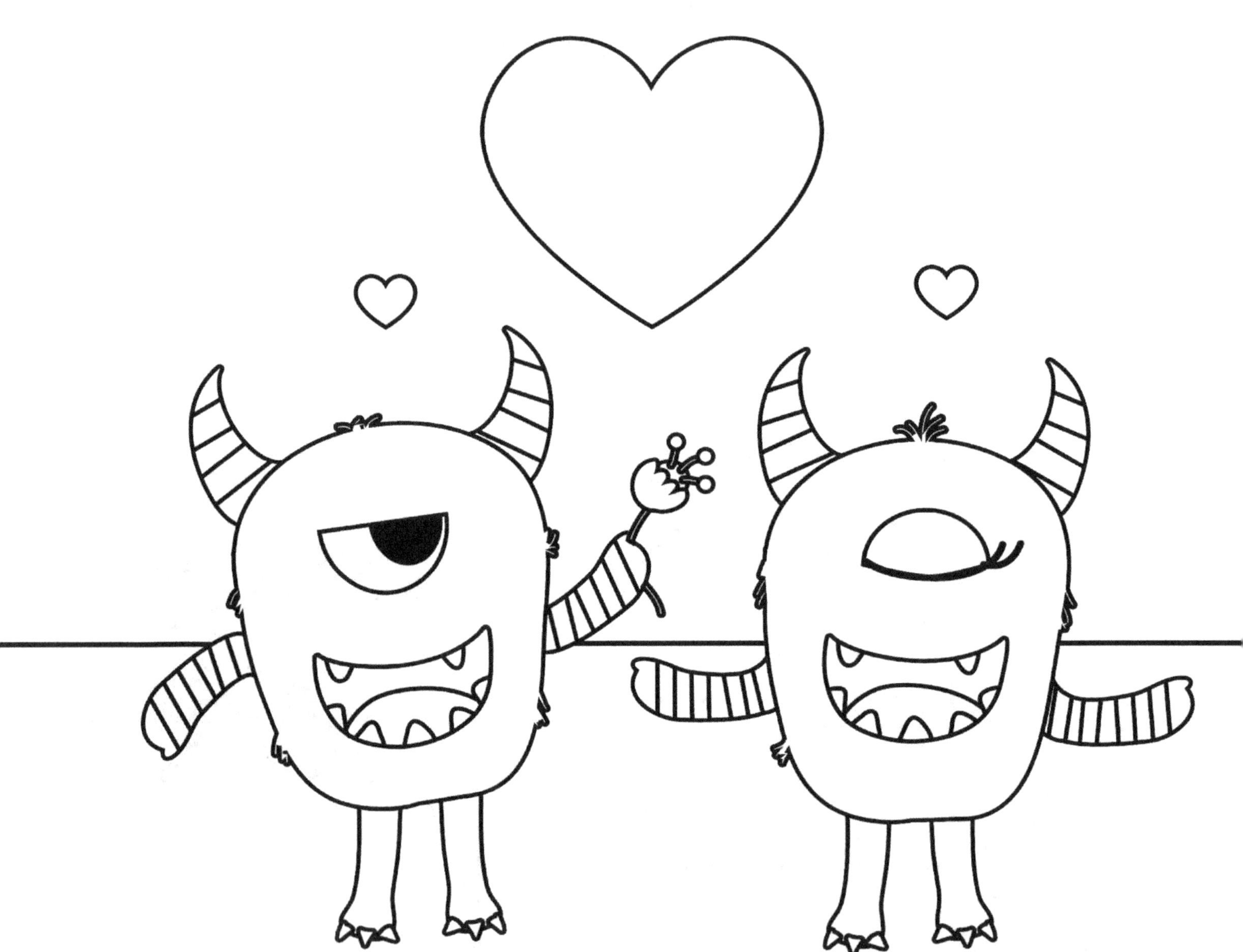

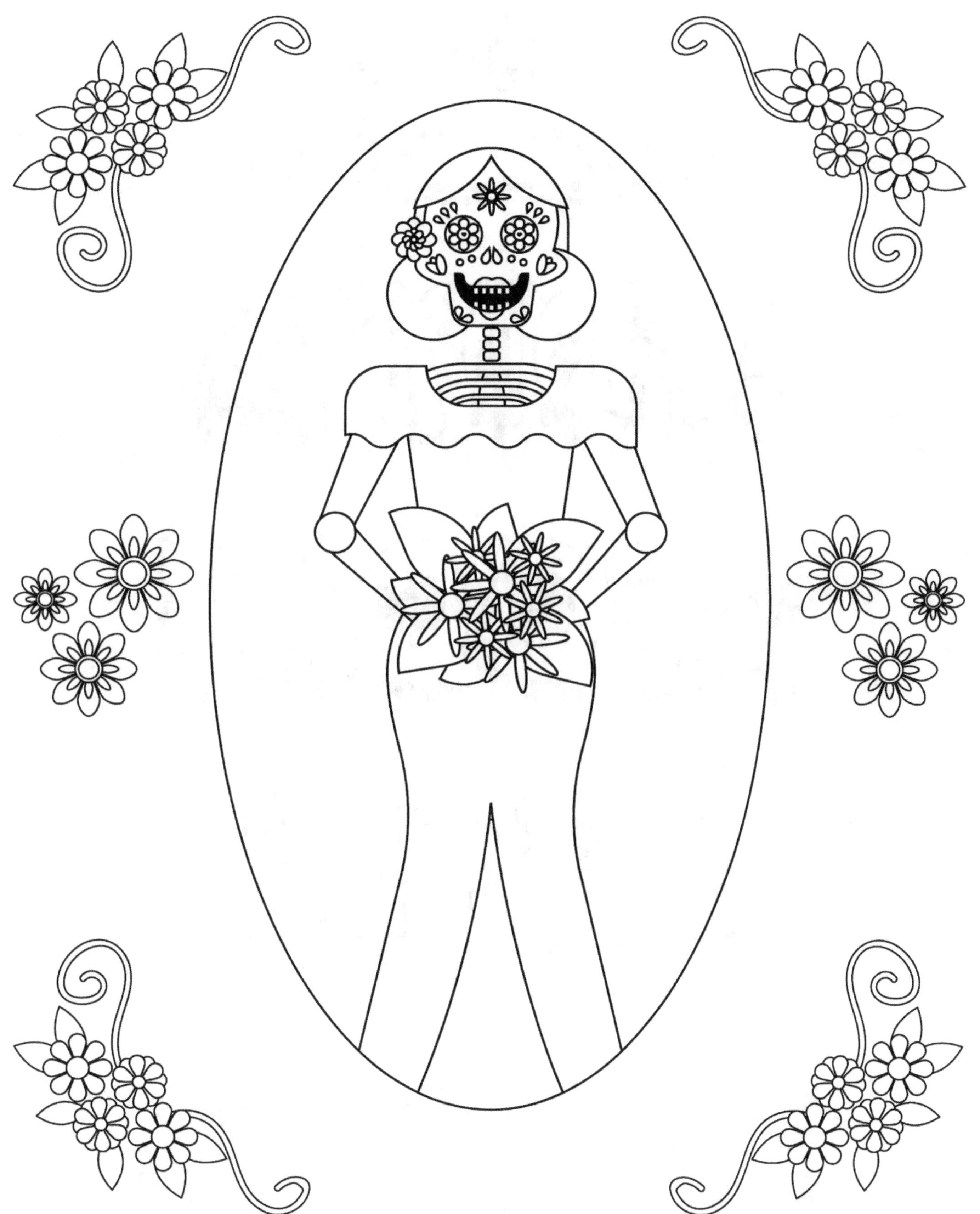

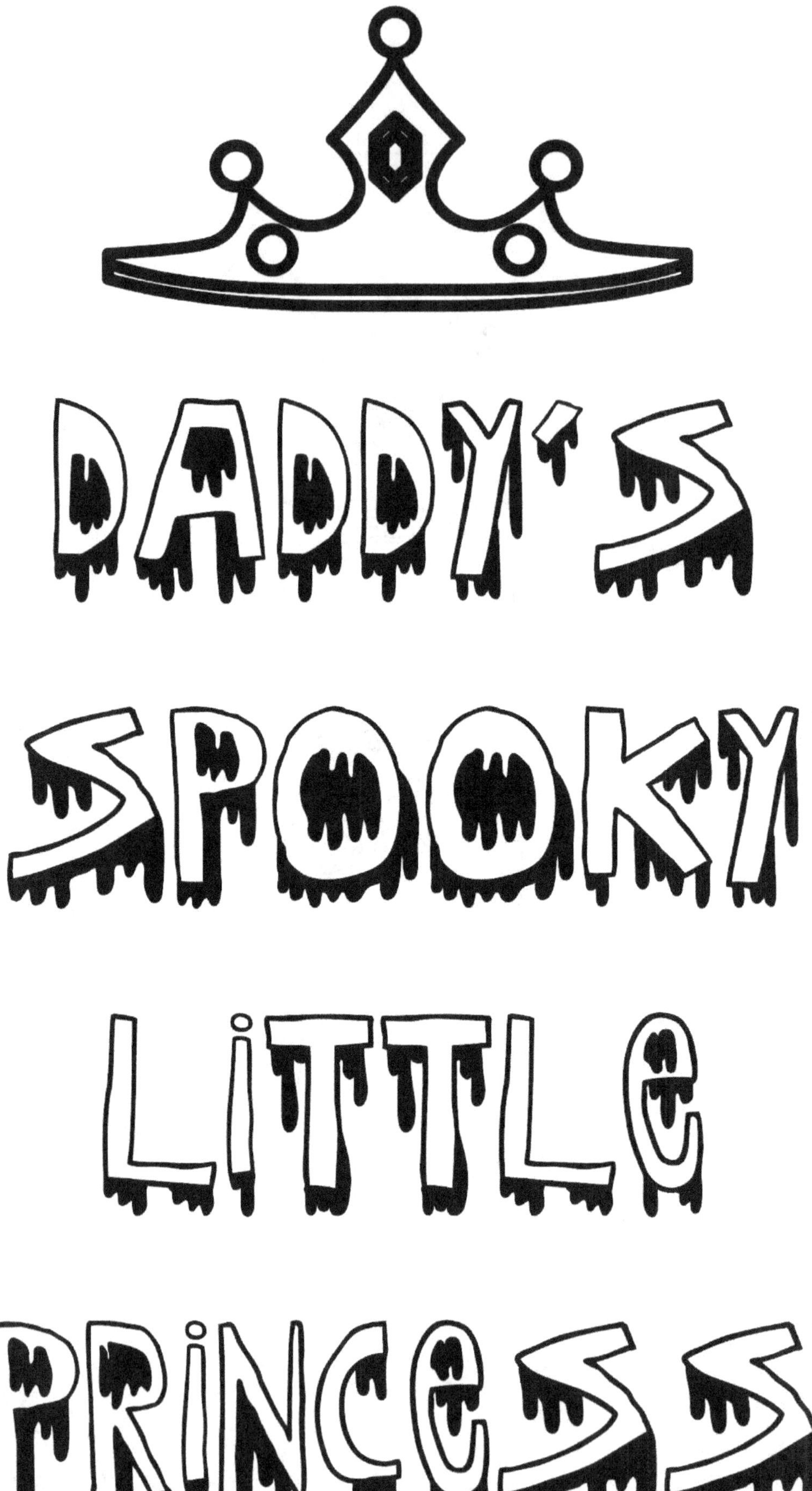
DADDY'S
SPOOKY
LITTLE
PRINCESS

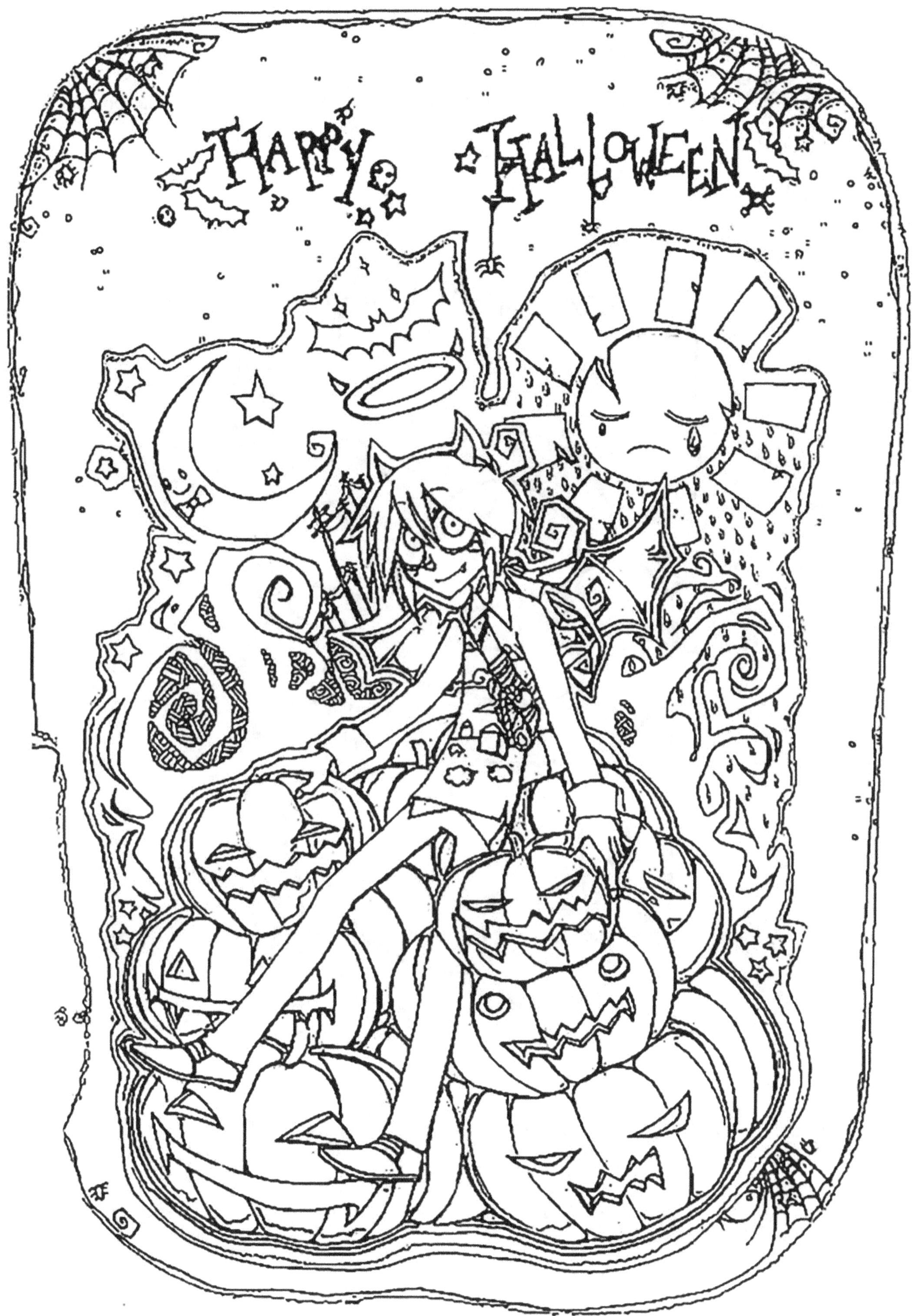

HAPPY HALLOWEEN

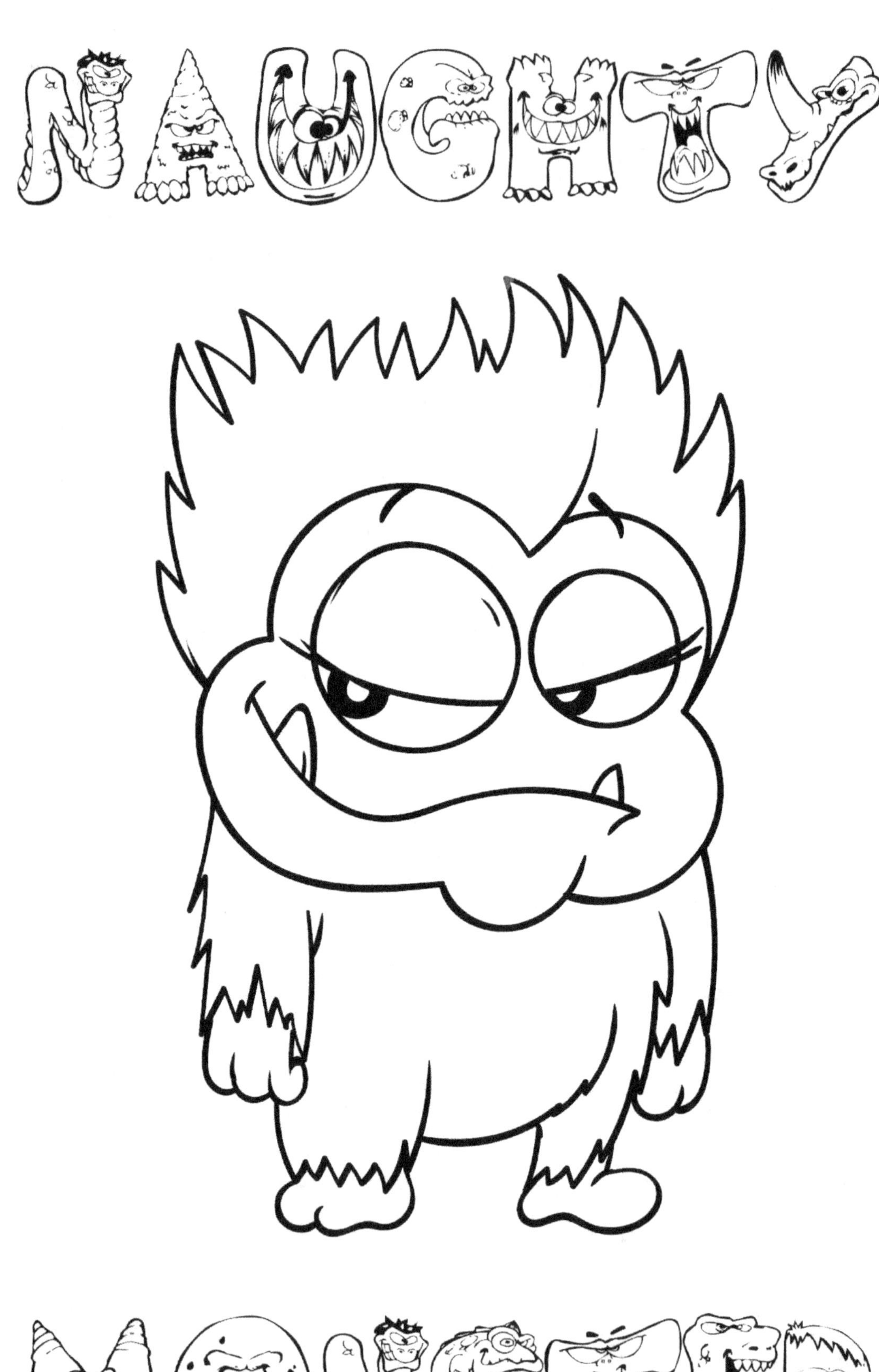

NAUGHTY
MONSTER

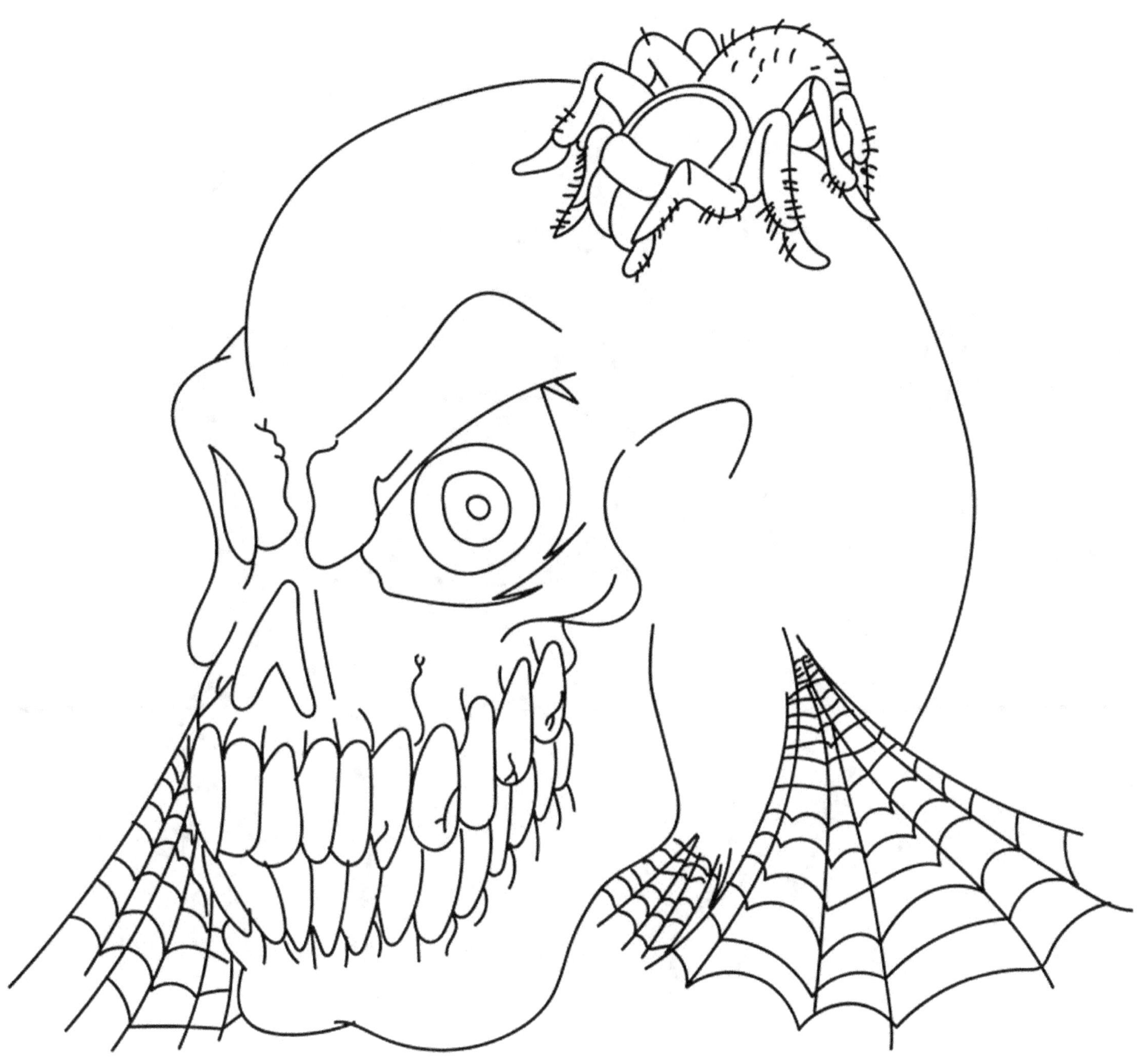

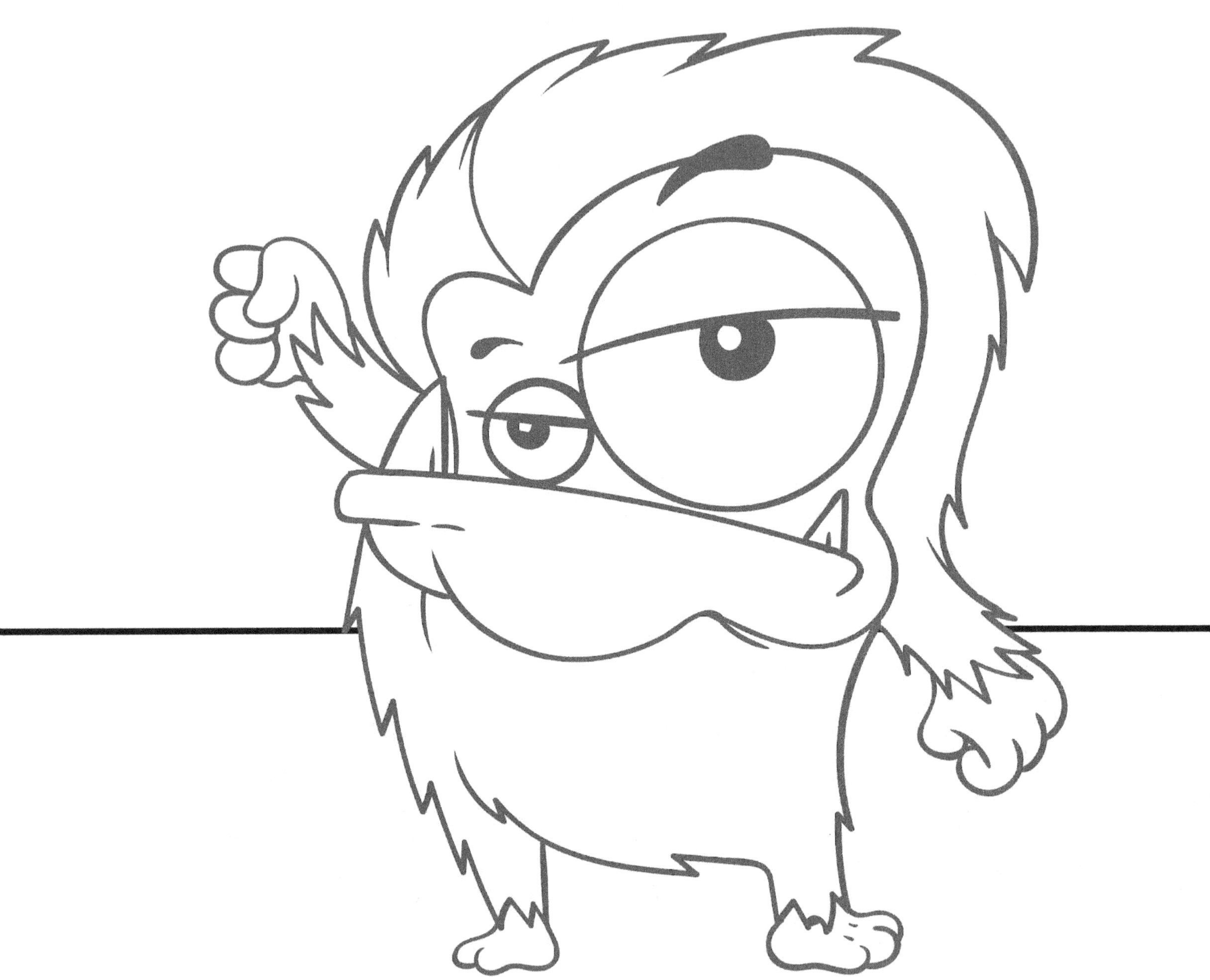

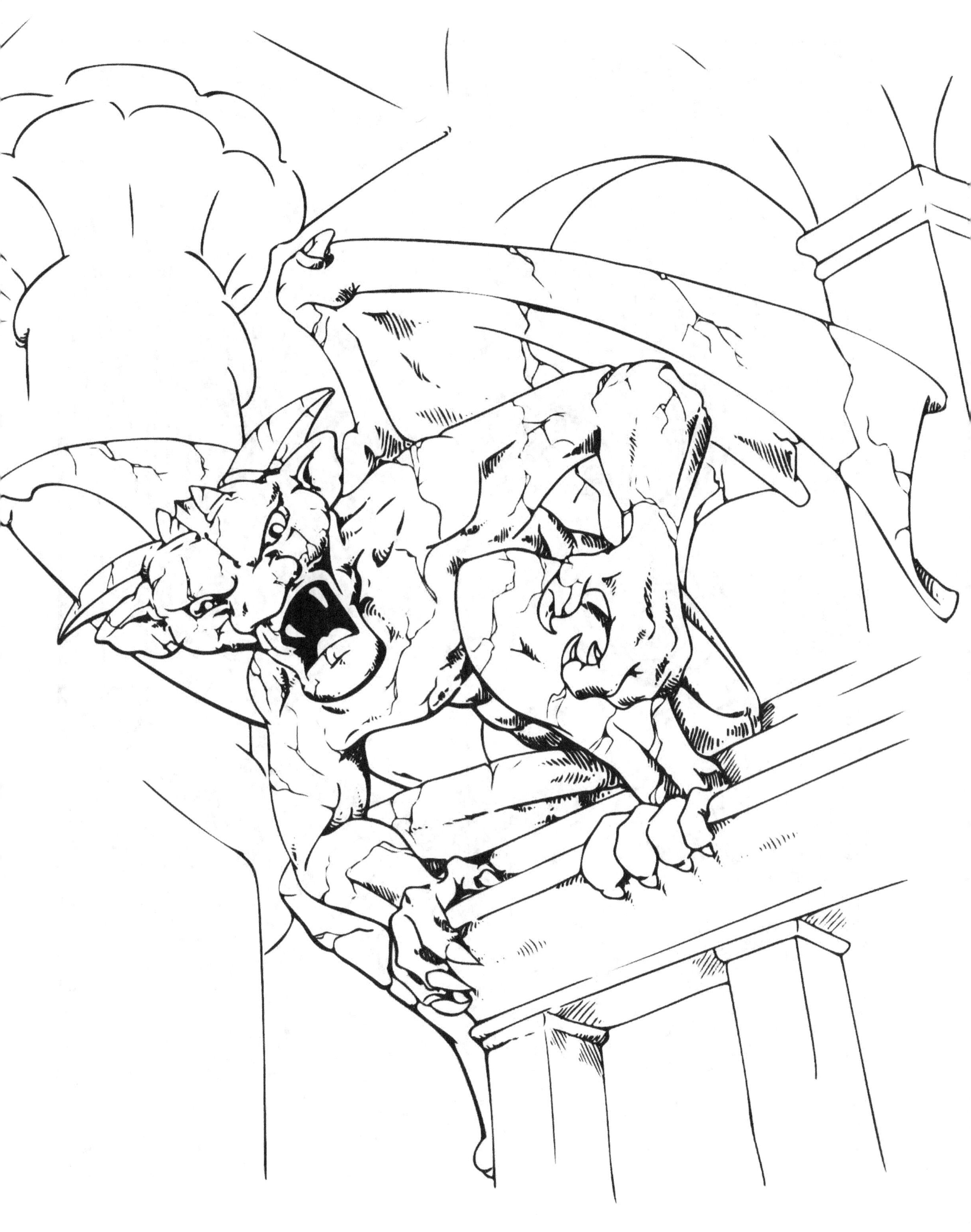

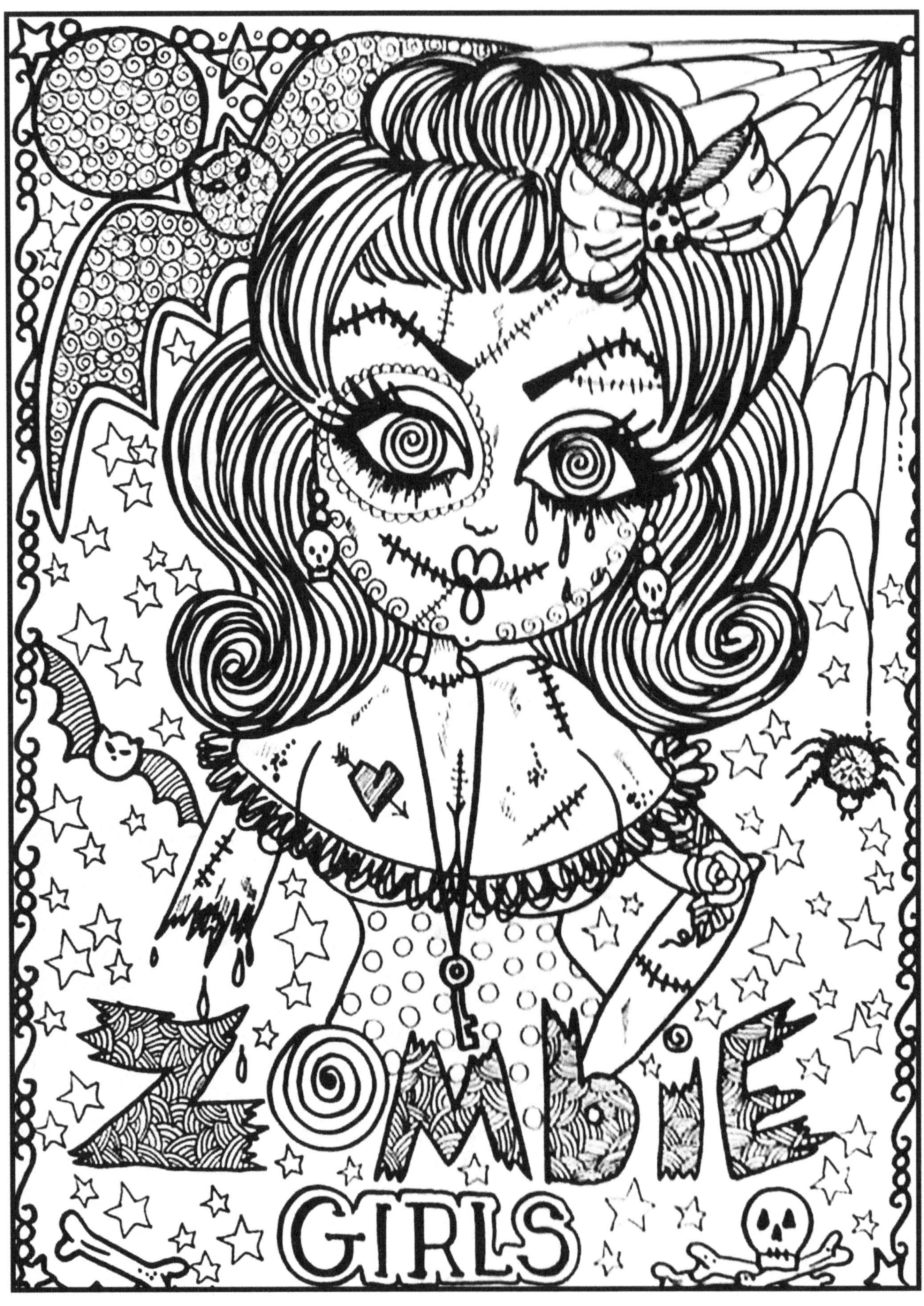

ZOMBIE
GIRLS

DADDYS CREEPY

LIL CUTIE

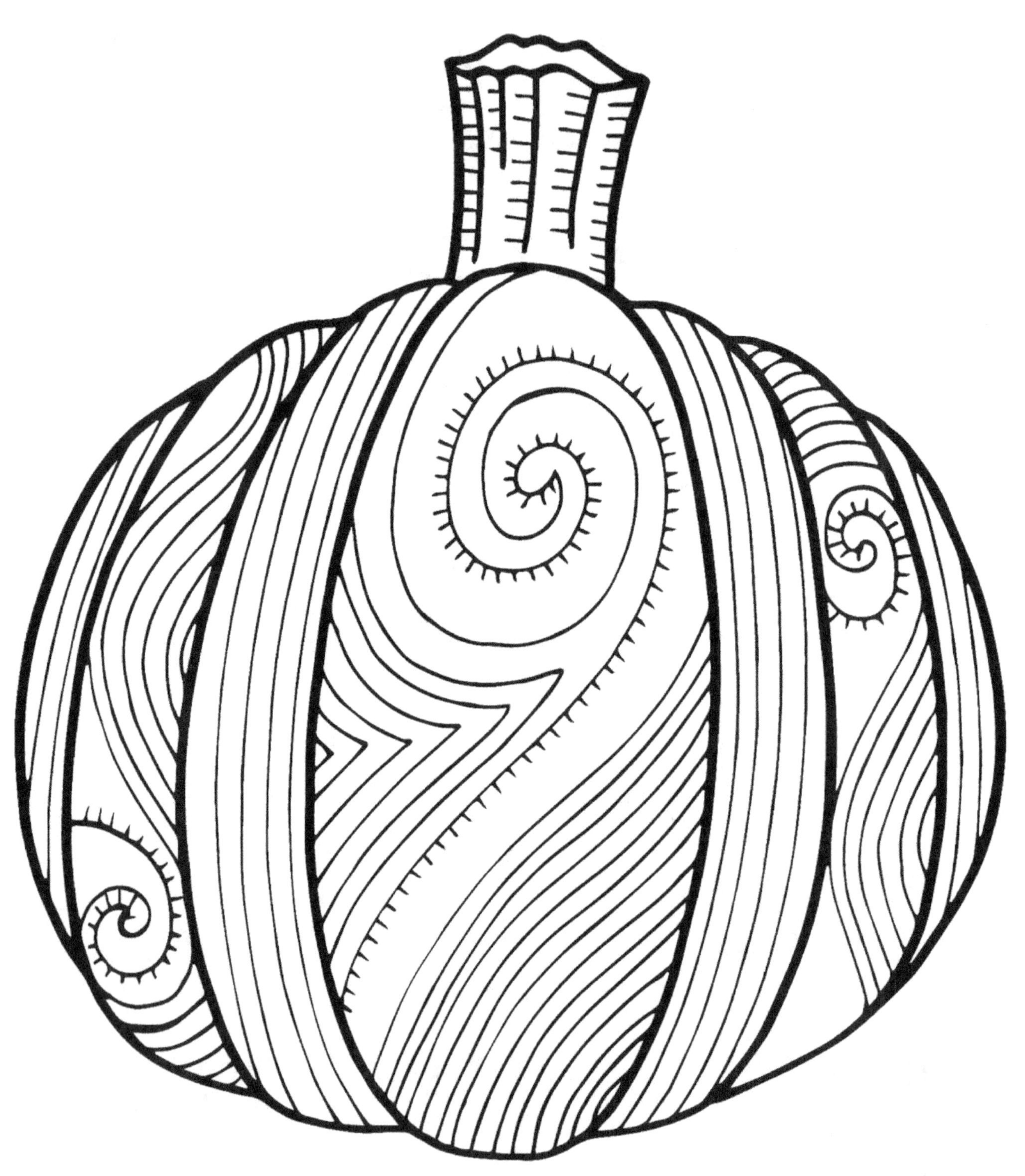

JUST GET ON YOUR KNEES AND BOB YOUR HEAD

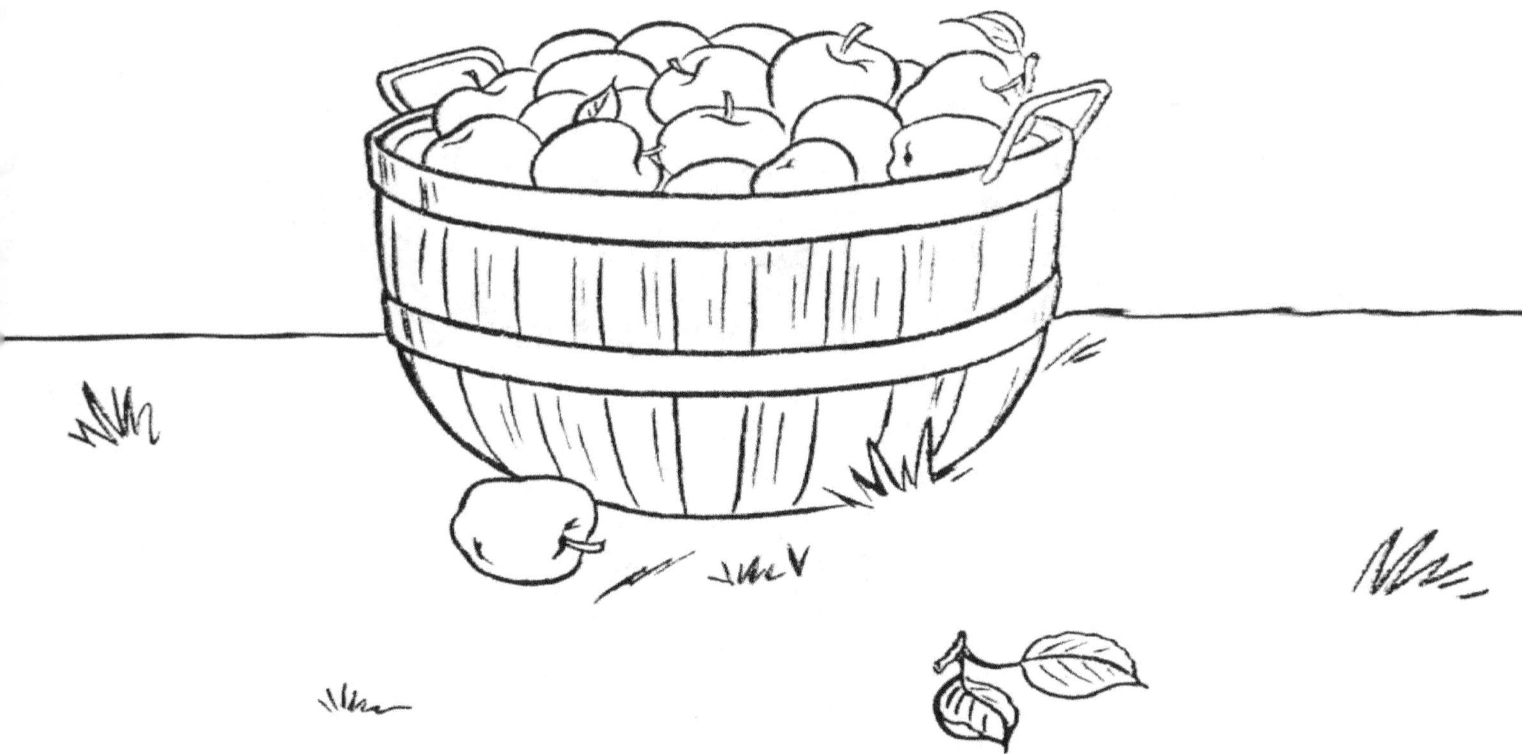

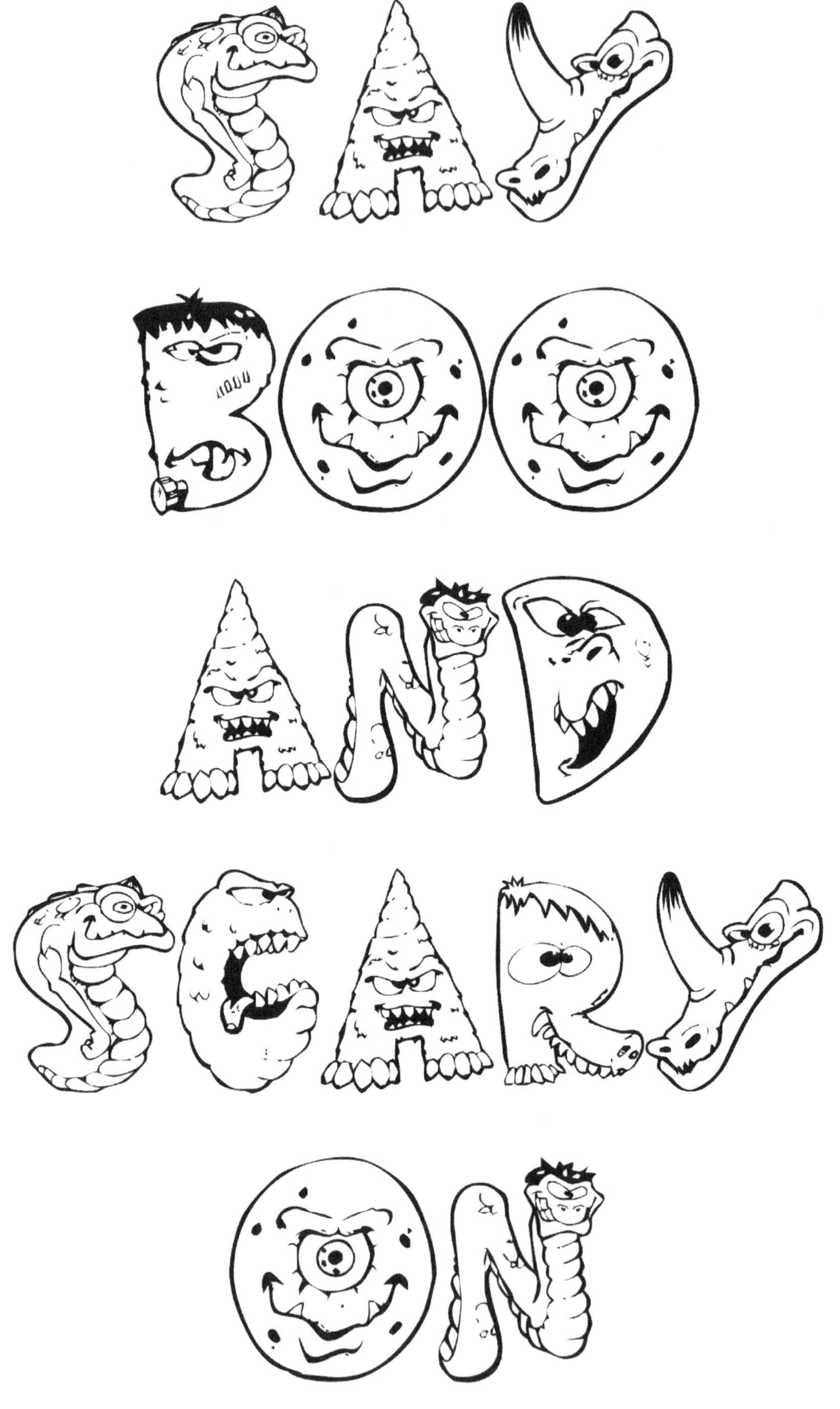

SAY
BOO
AND
SCARY
ON

HELP THE DADDY ZOMBIE FIND HIS LITTLE ONE!

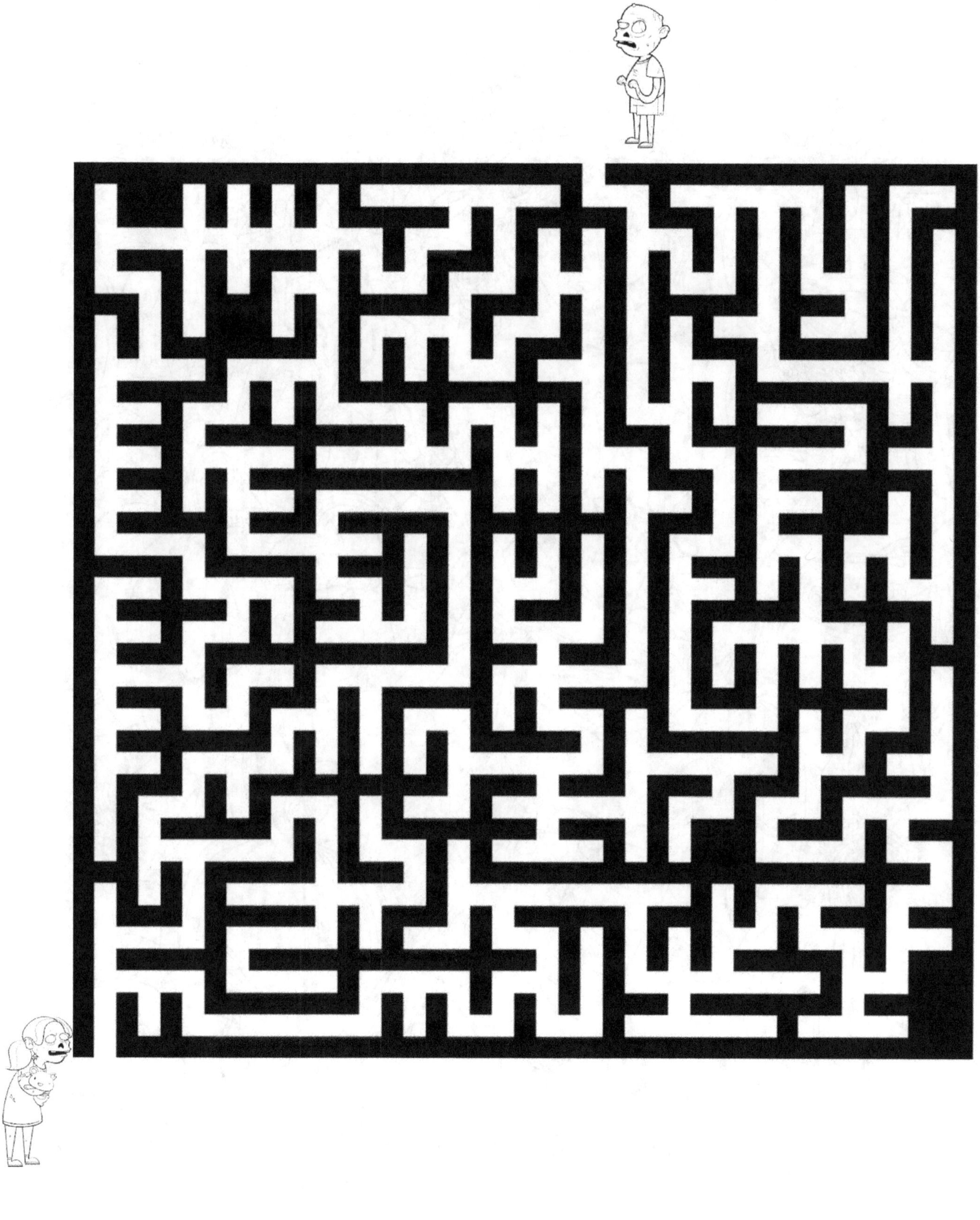

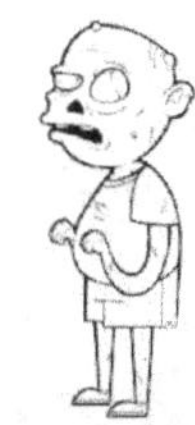

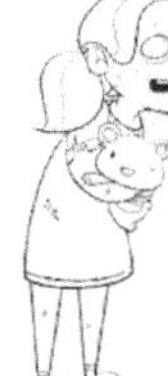

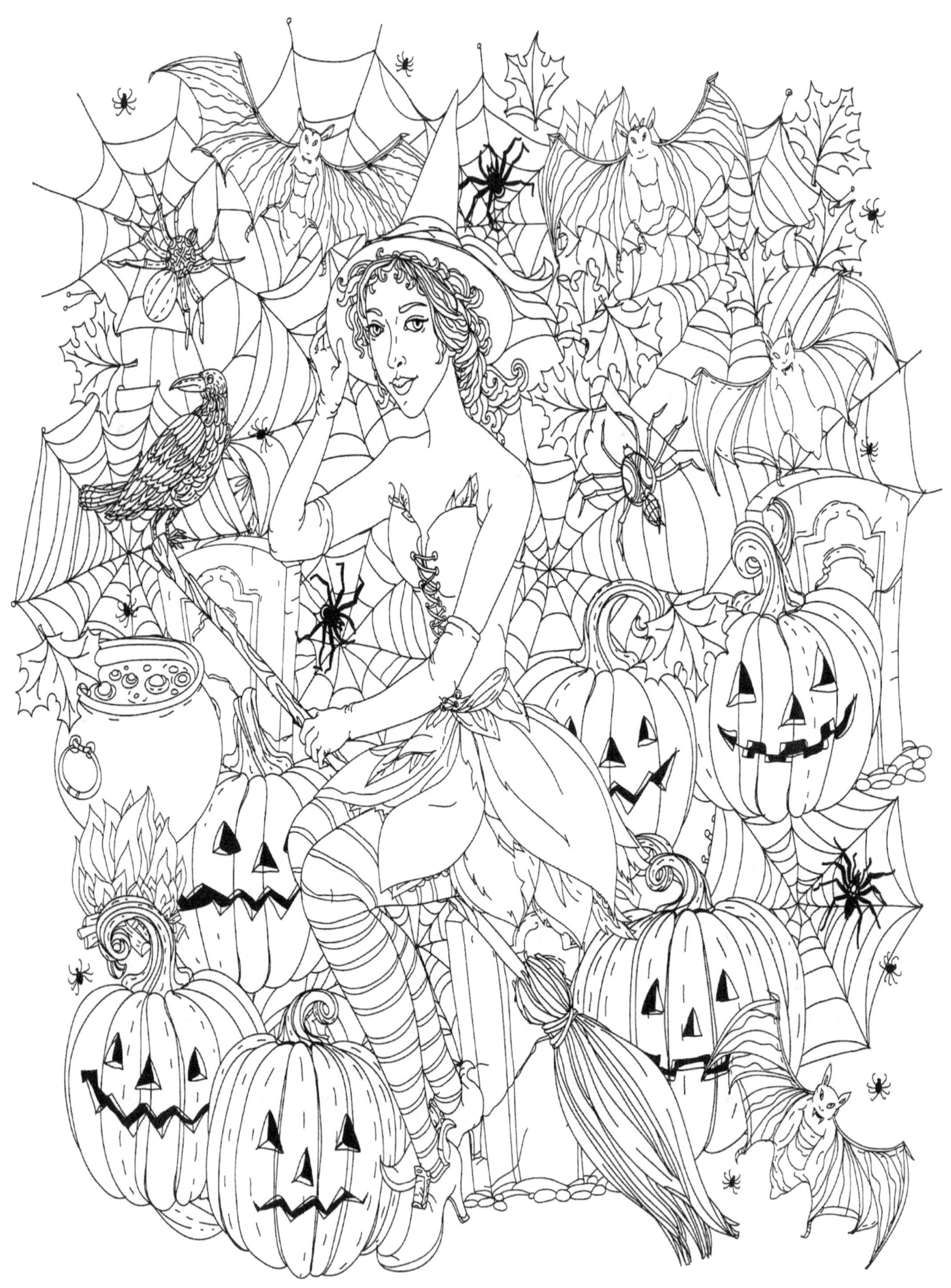

DECORATE THE SPOOKY MASKS, THEN CUT THEM OUT TO WEAR!

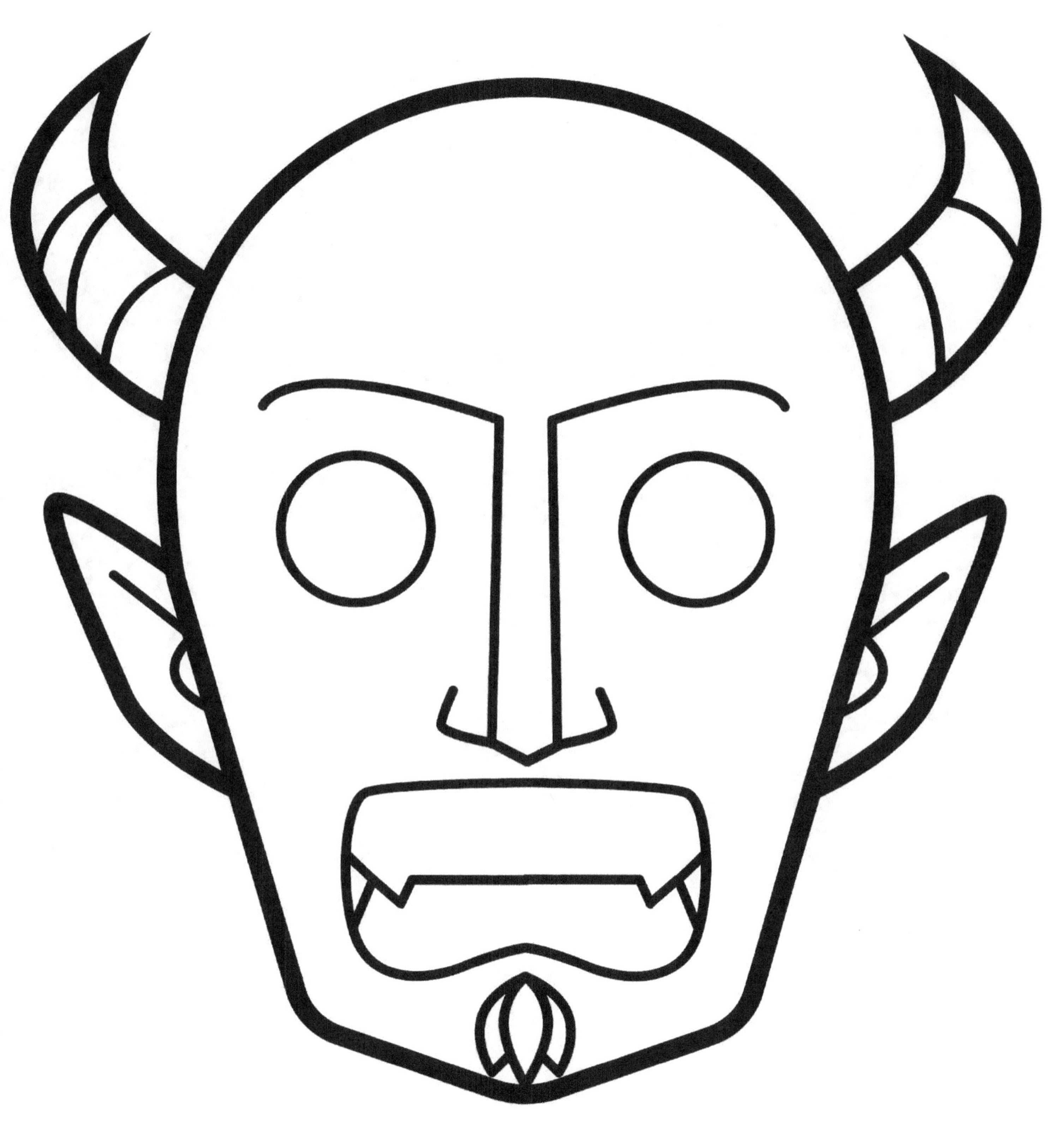

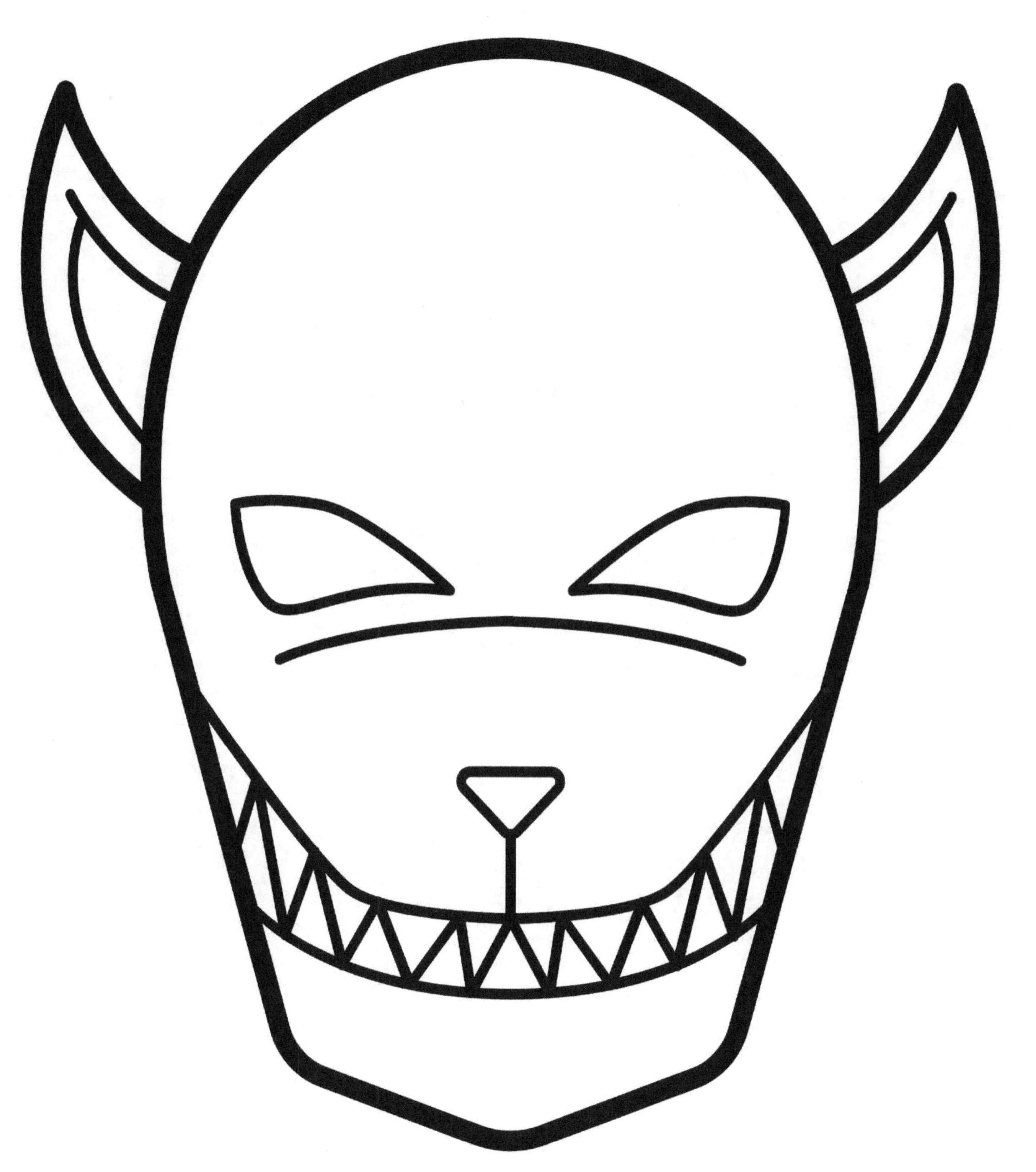

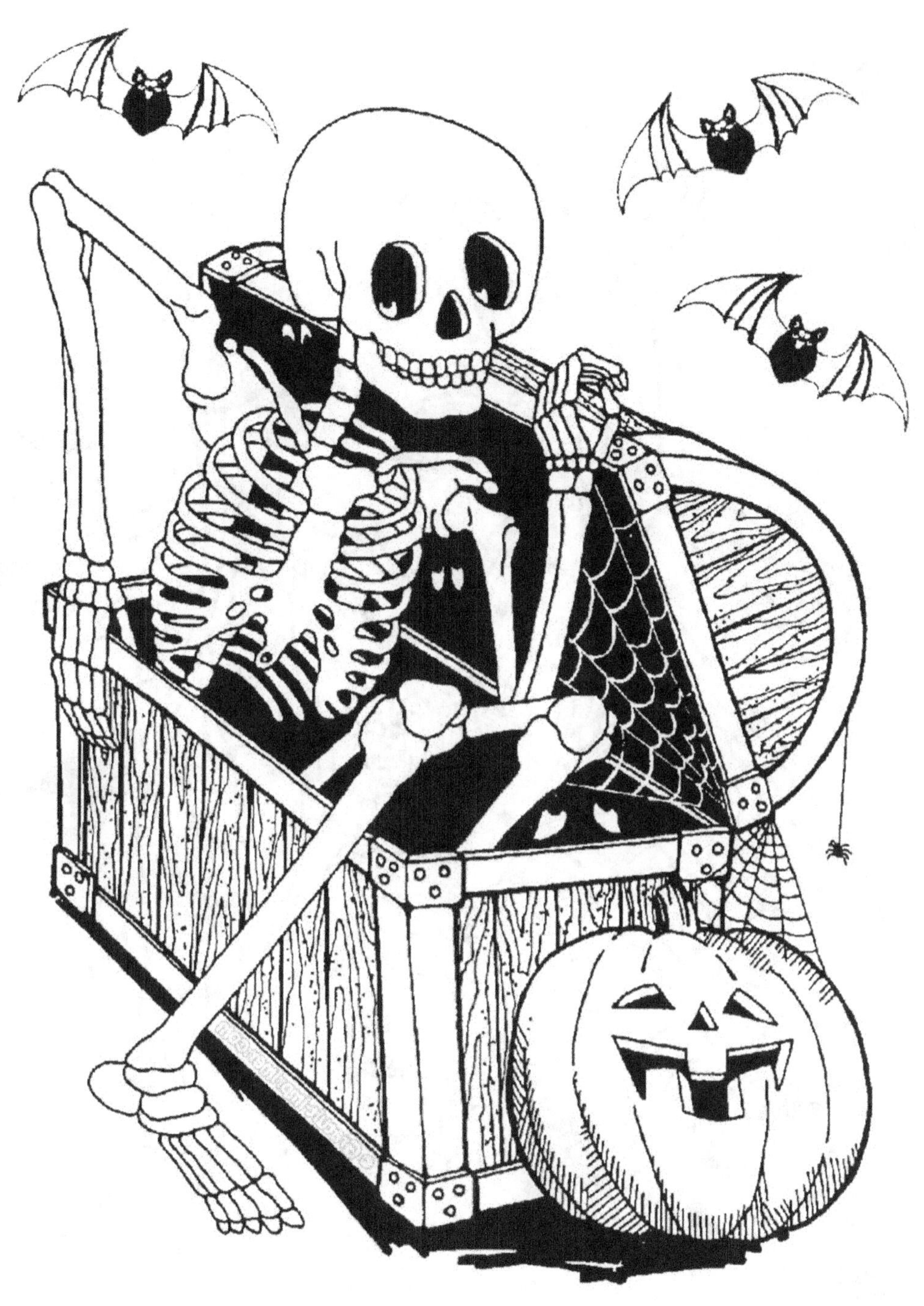

BONE DADDY

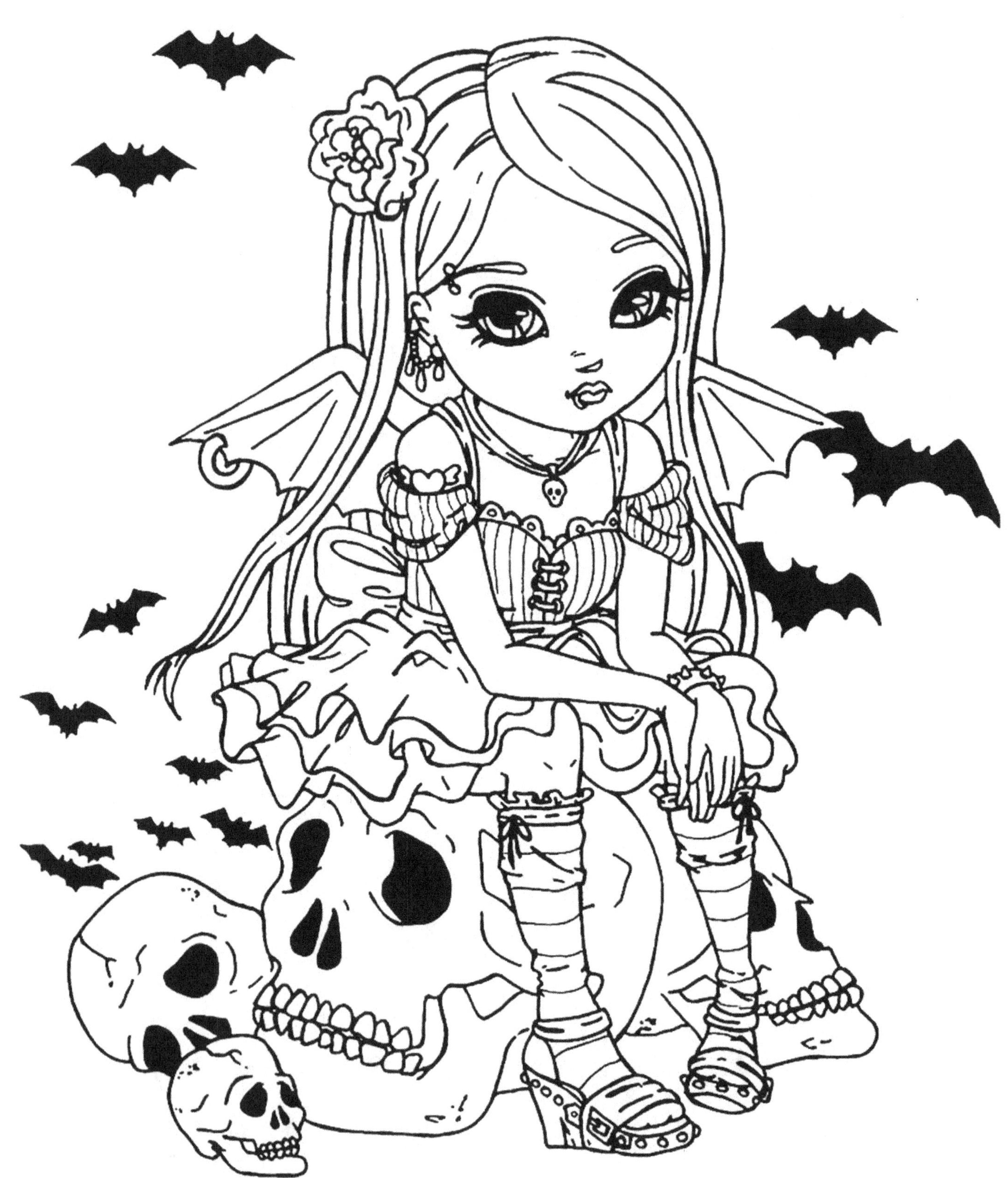

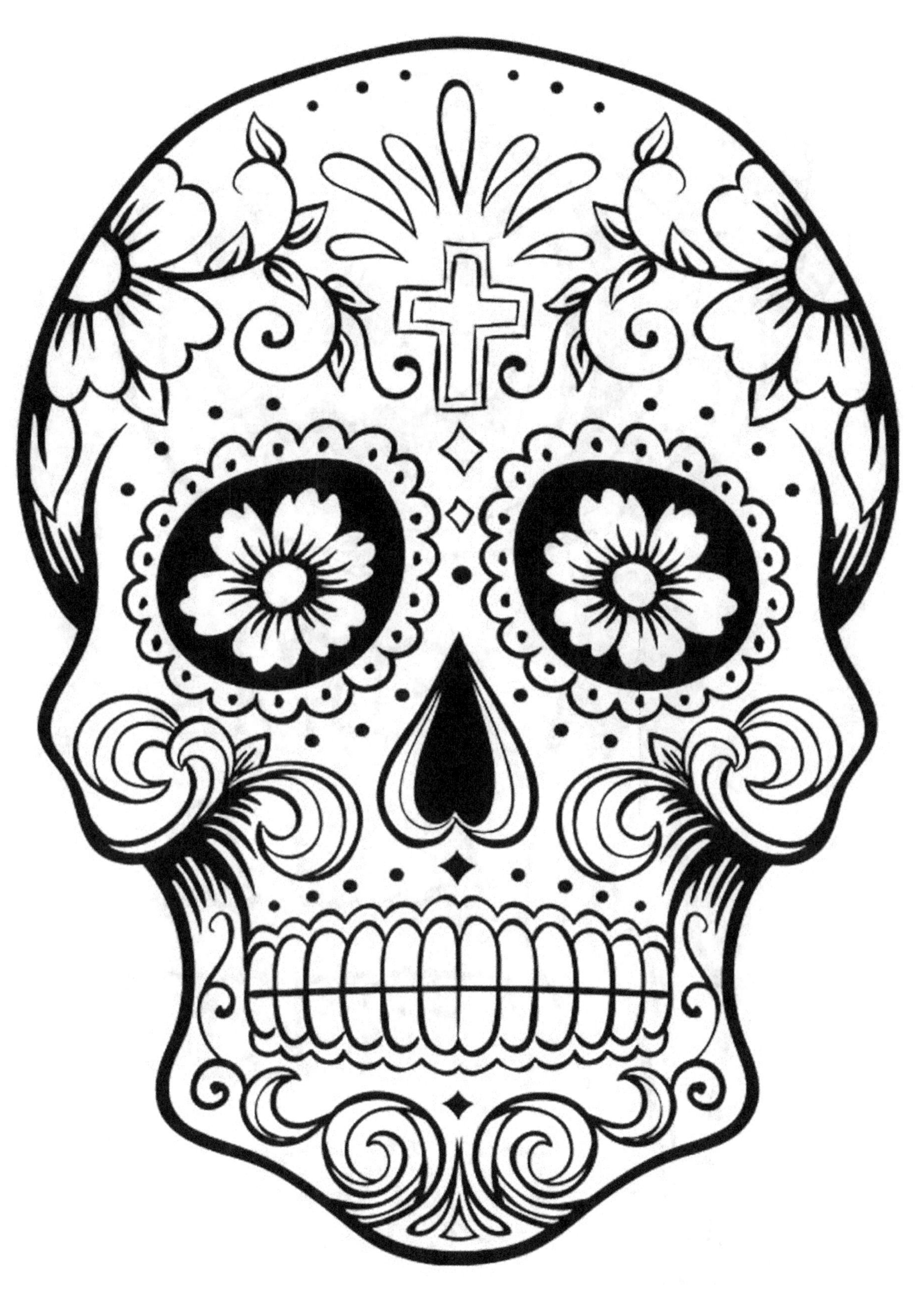

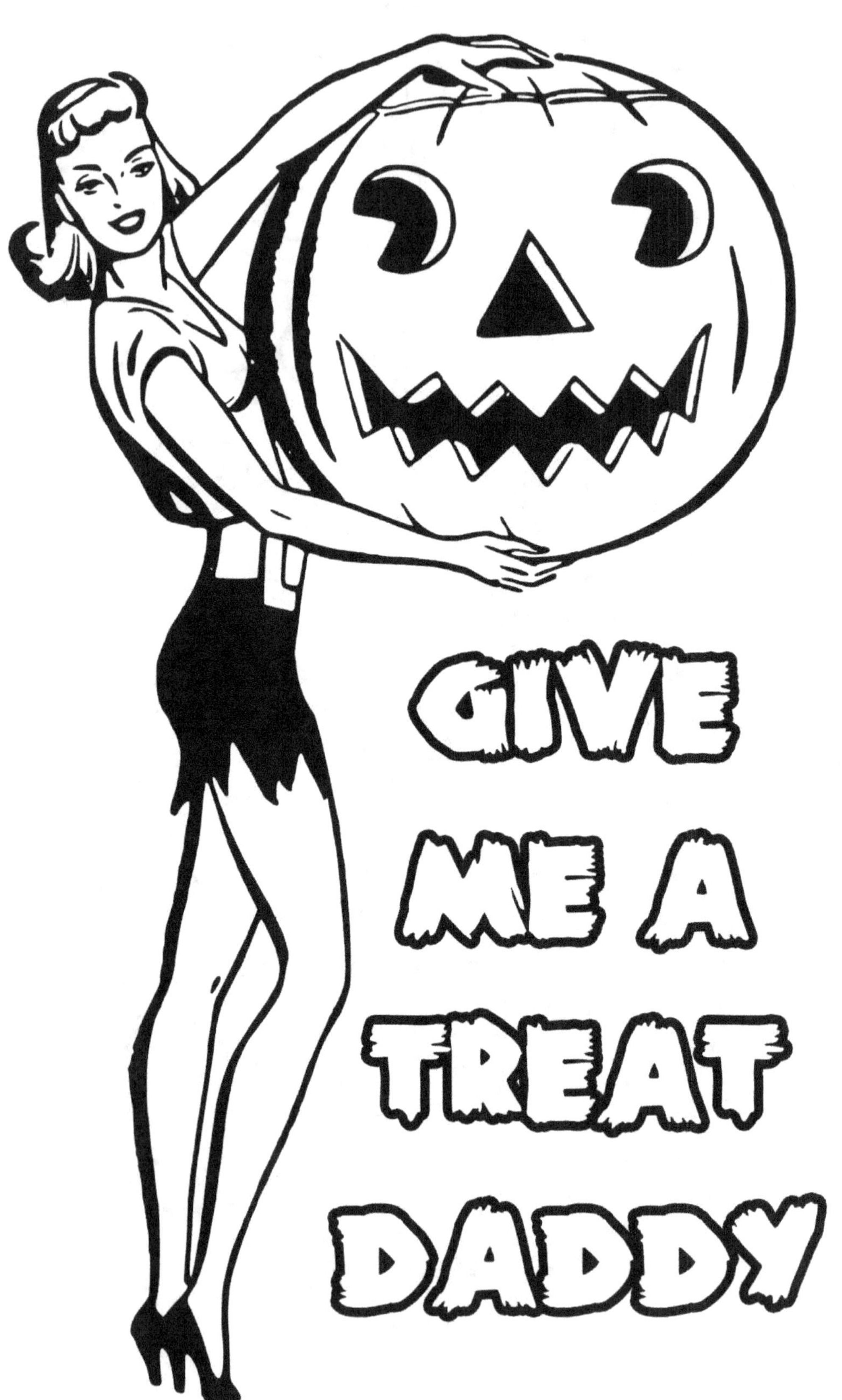
GIVE
ME A
TREAT
DADDY

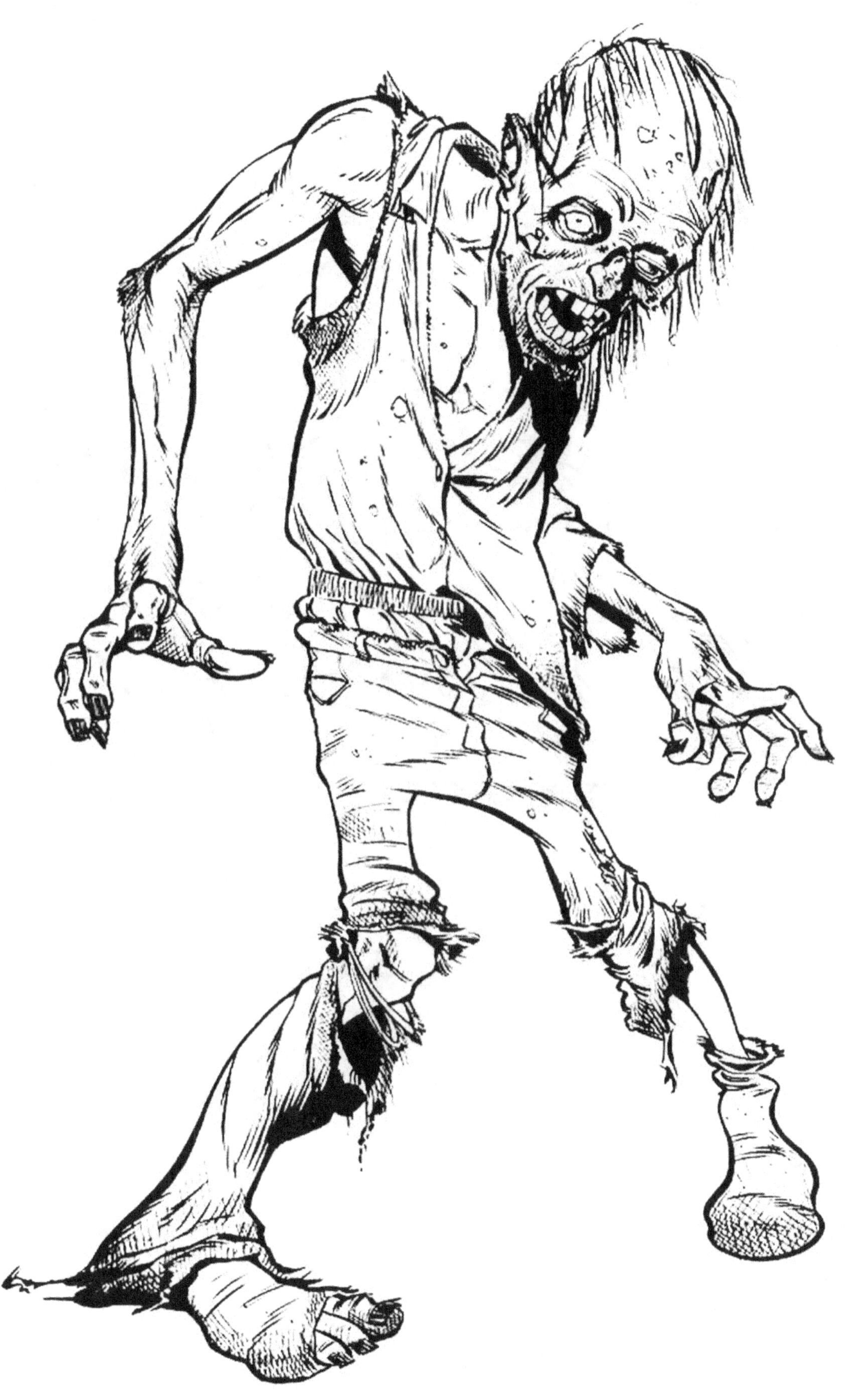

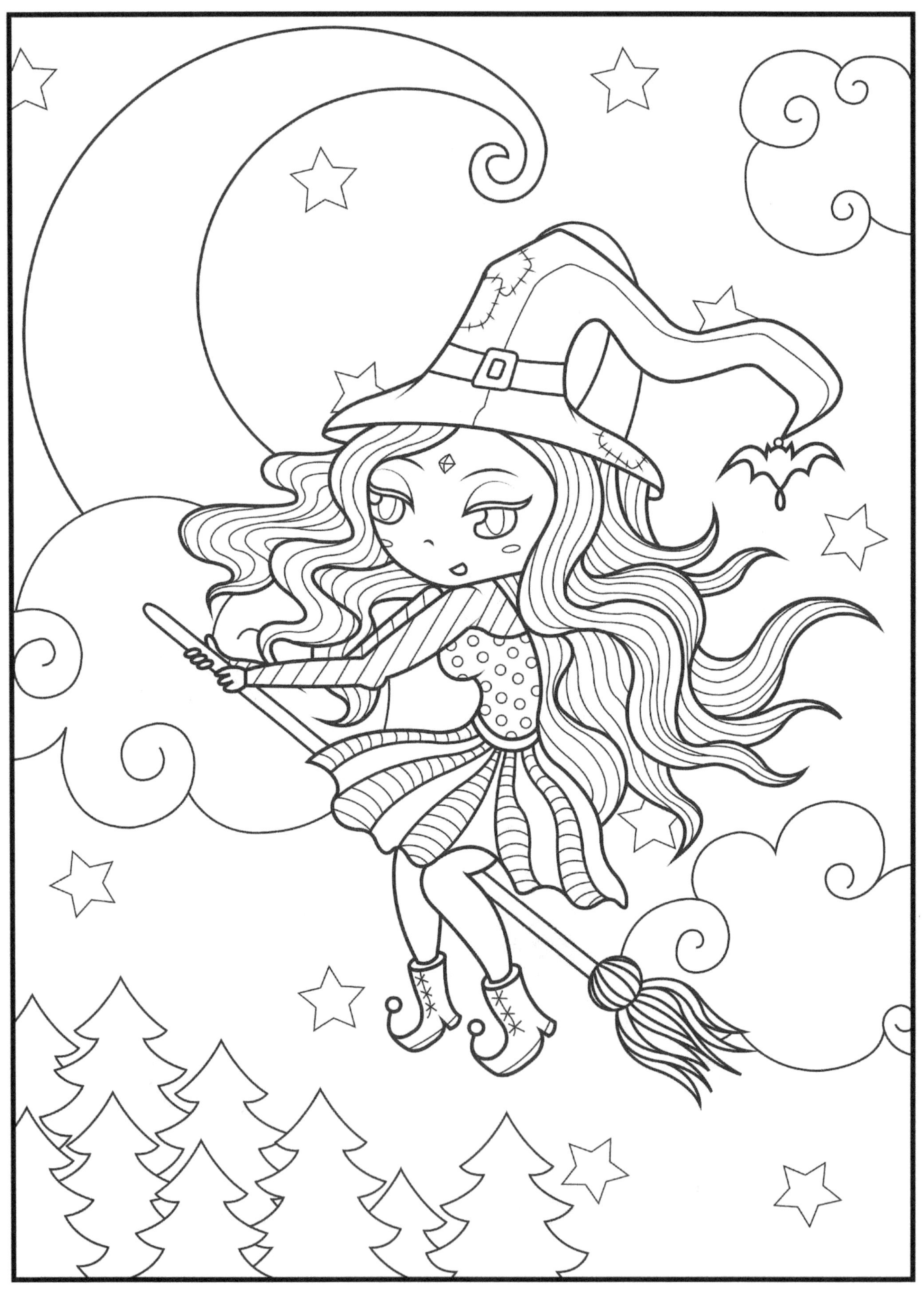

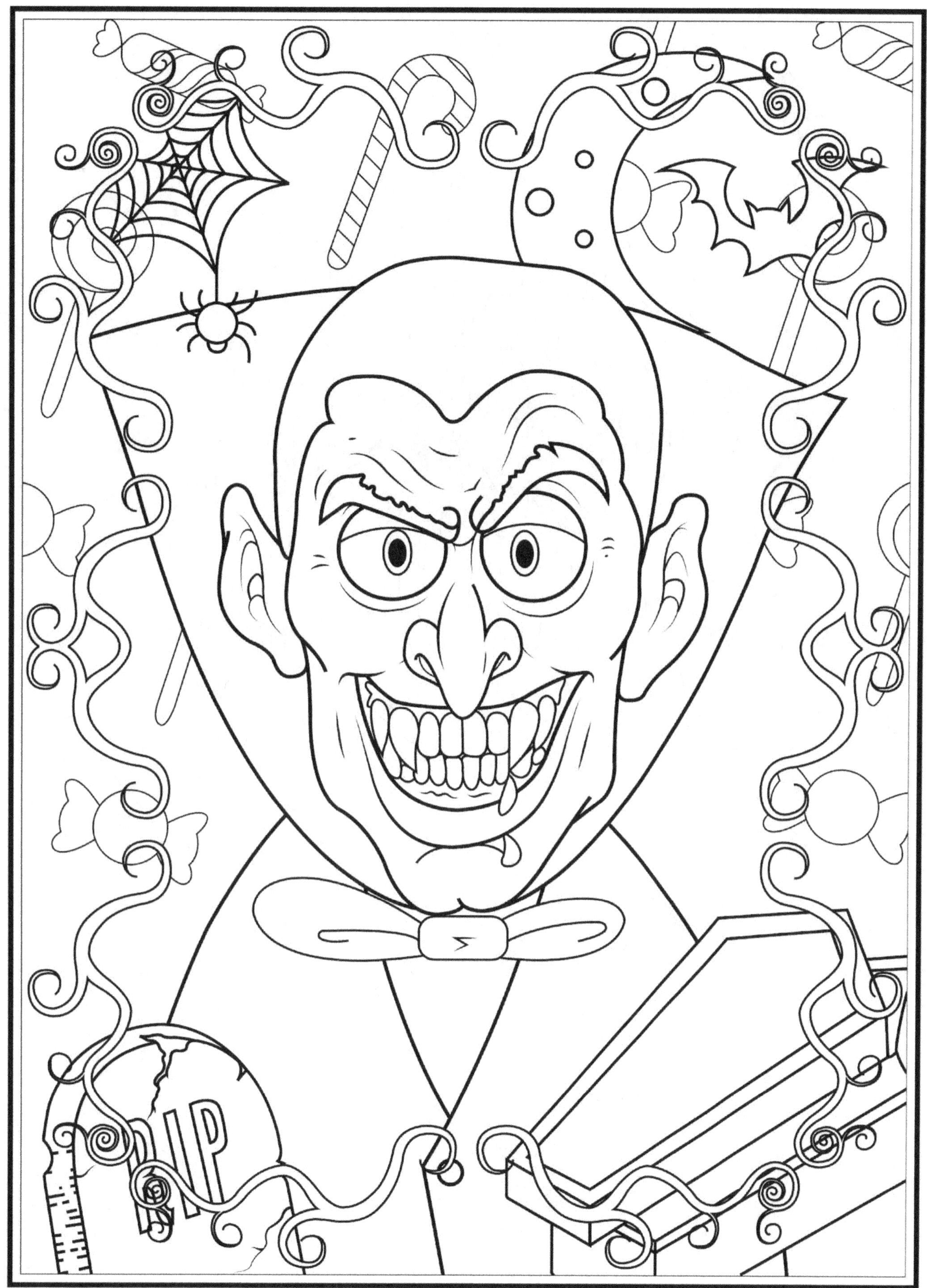

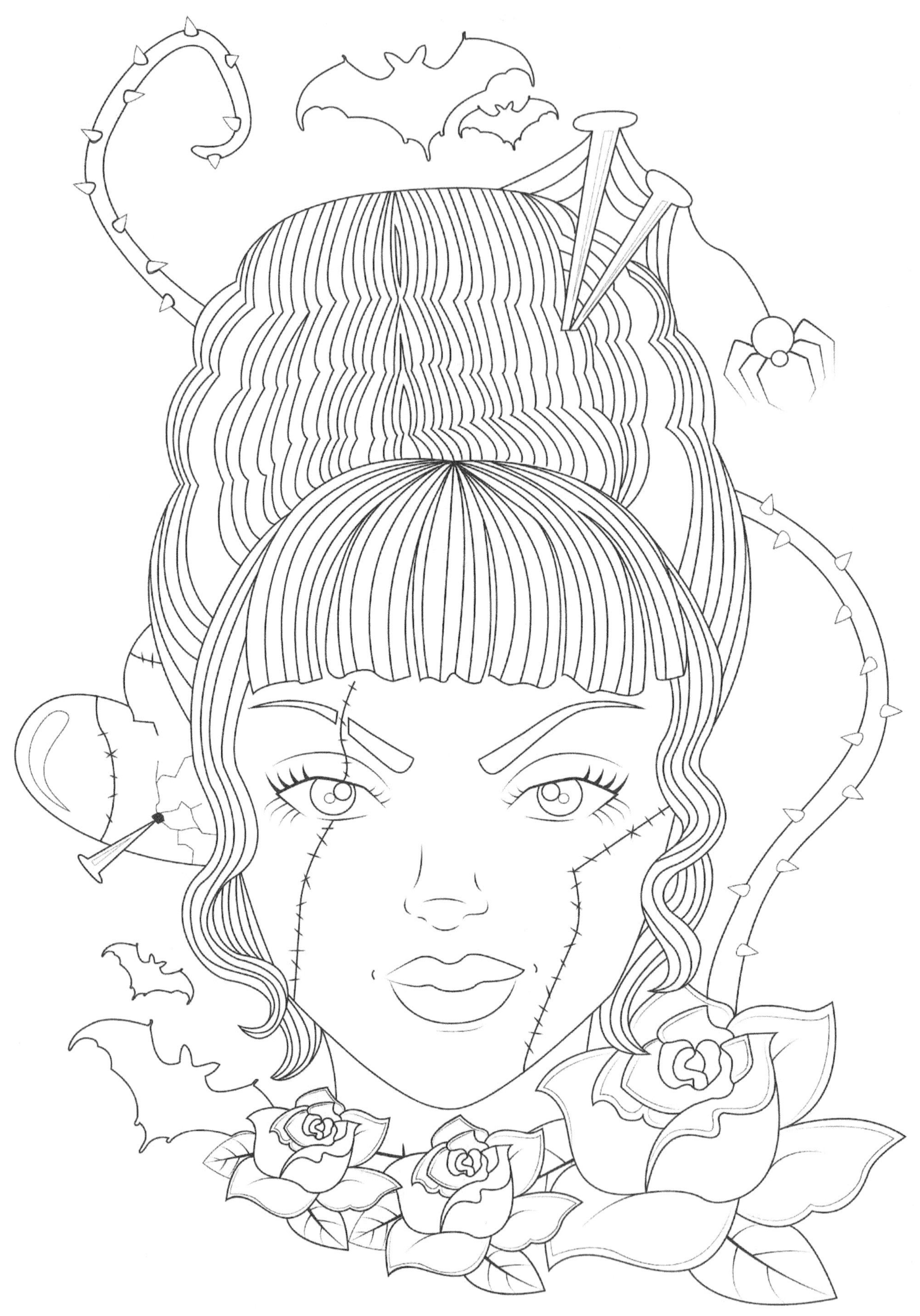

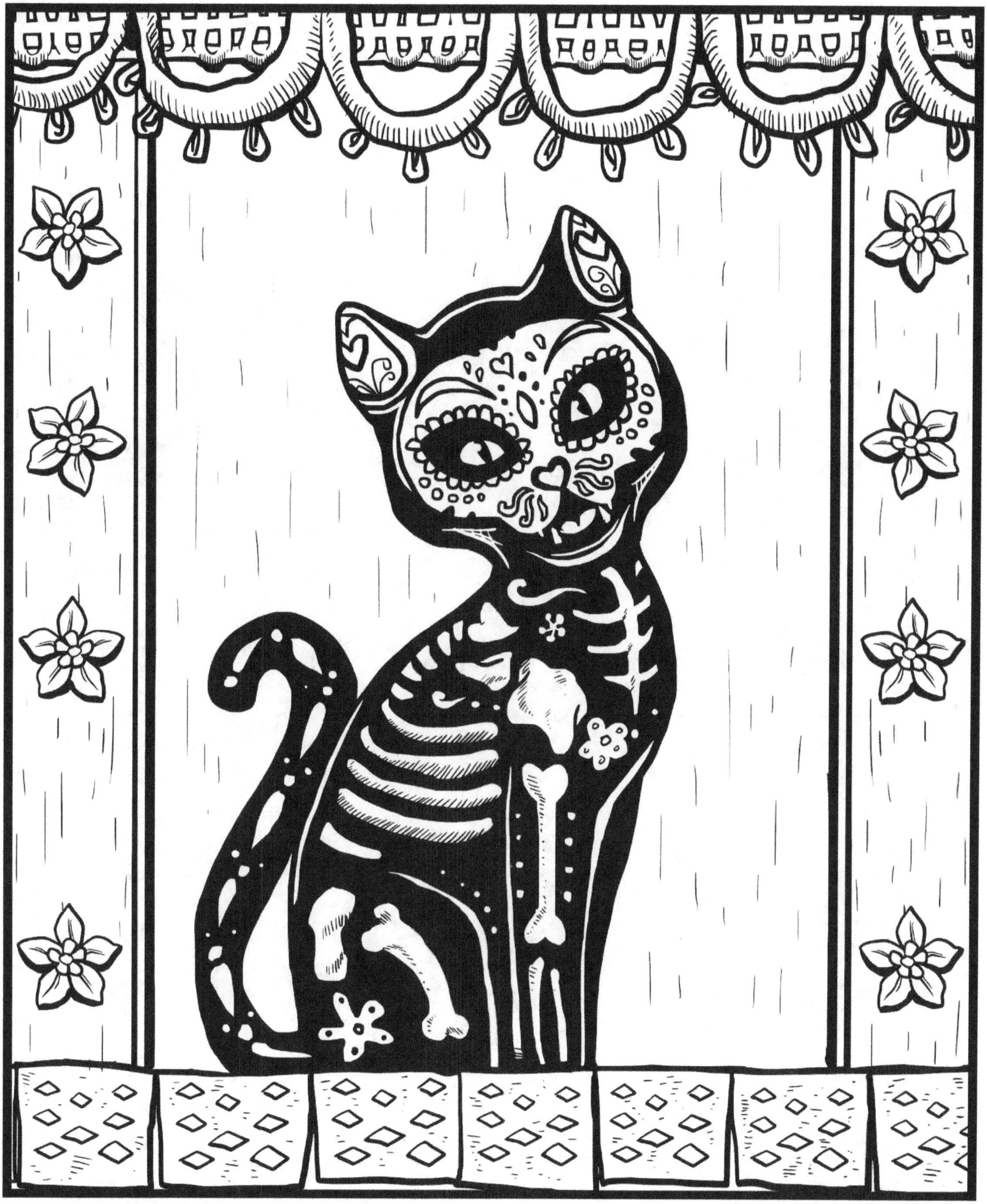

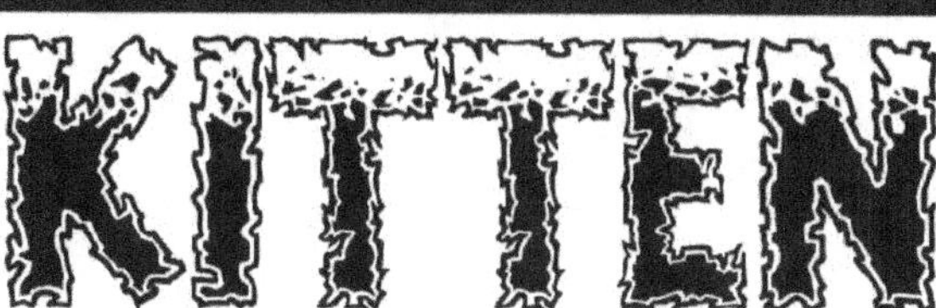

SPOOKY KITTEN

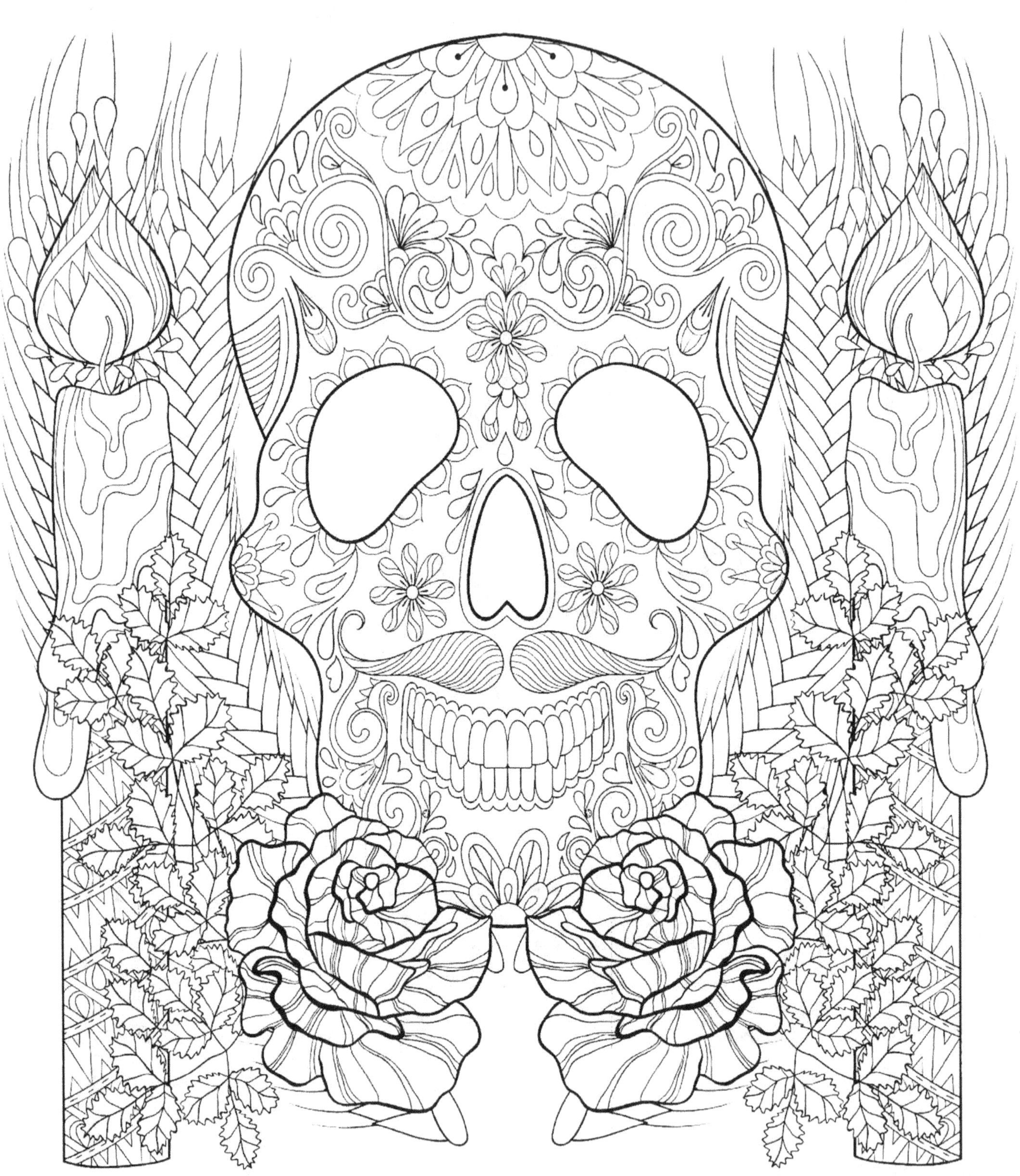

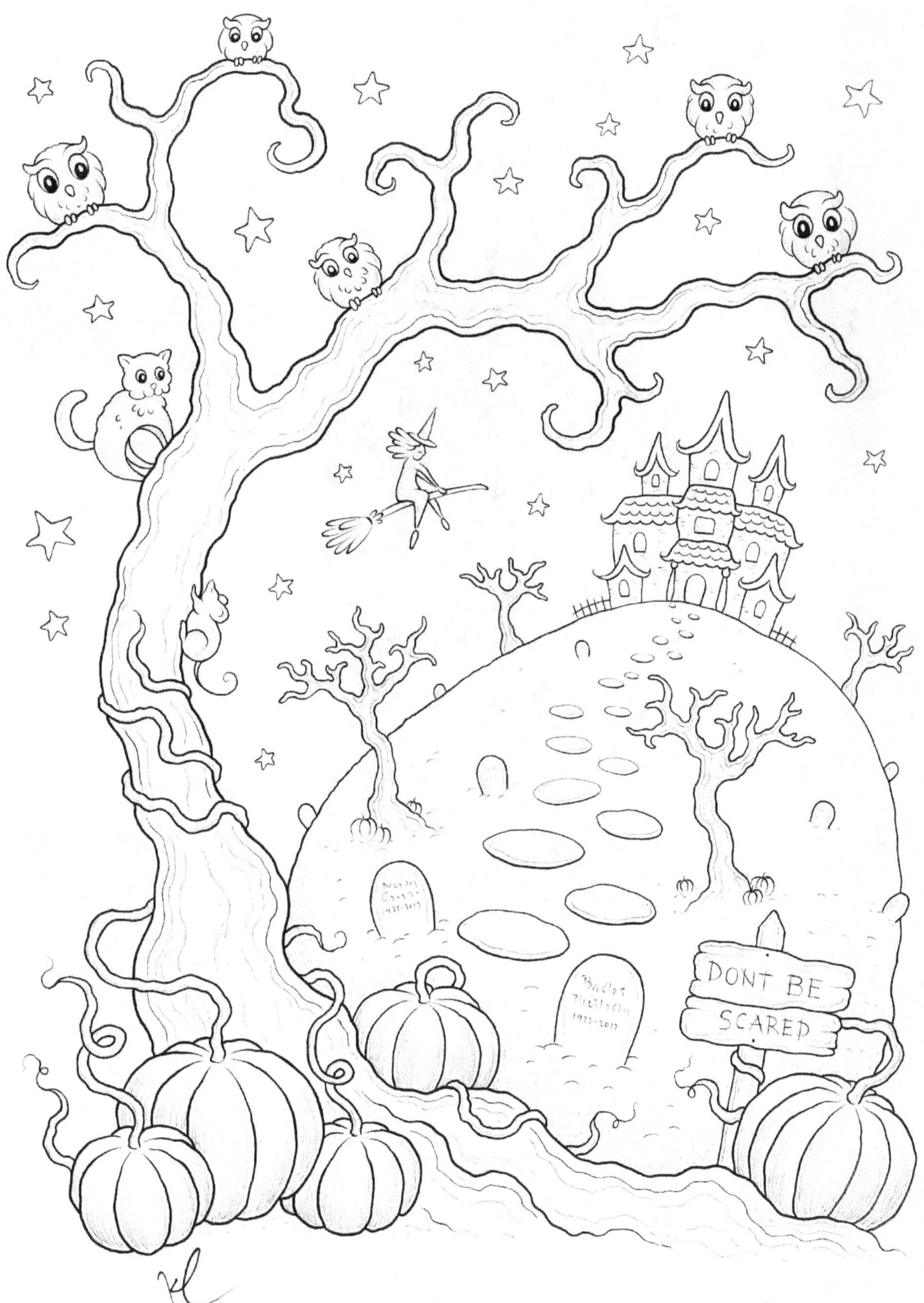
DONT BE SCARED

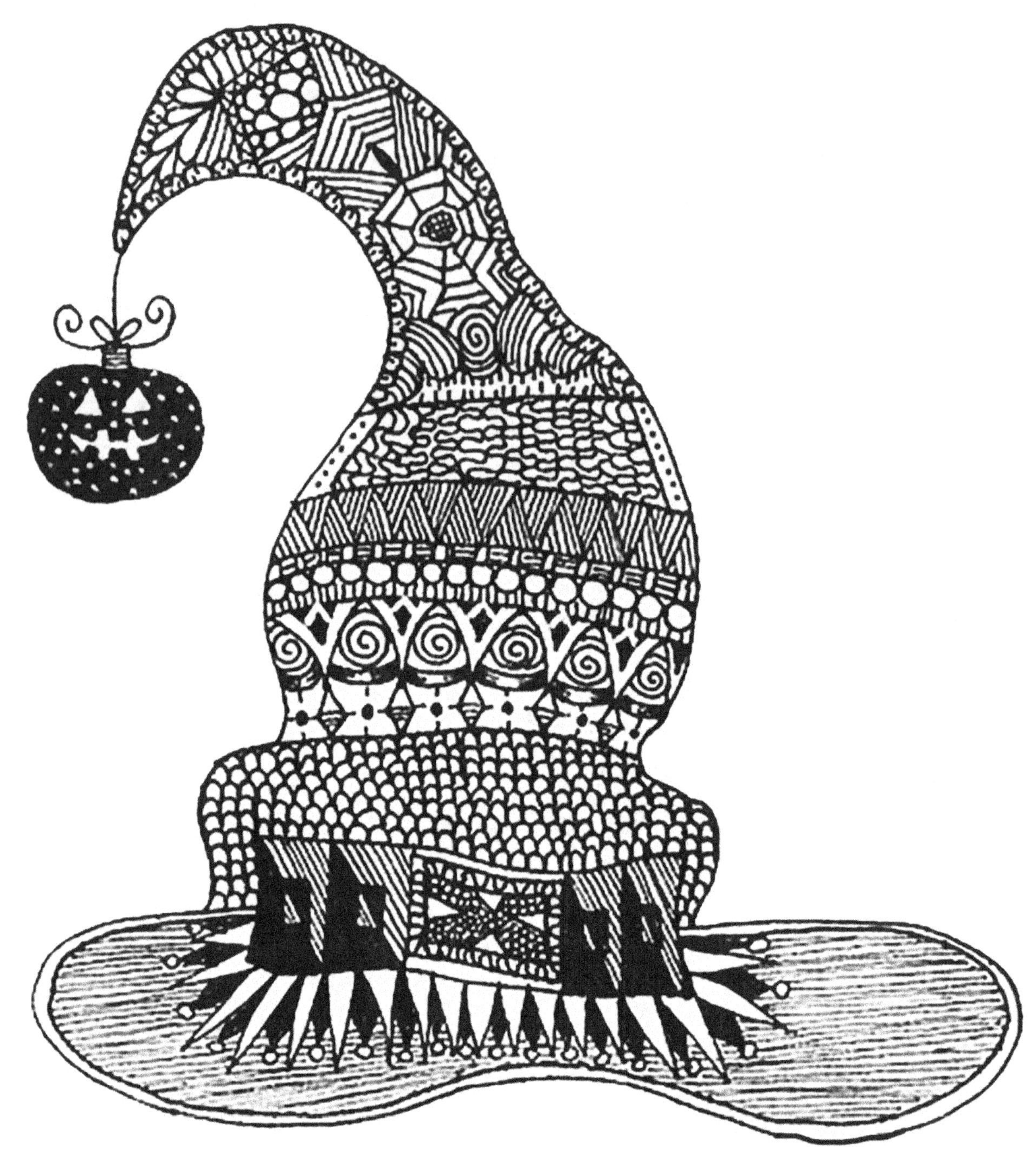

FEELING WITCHY

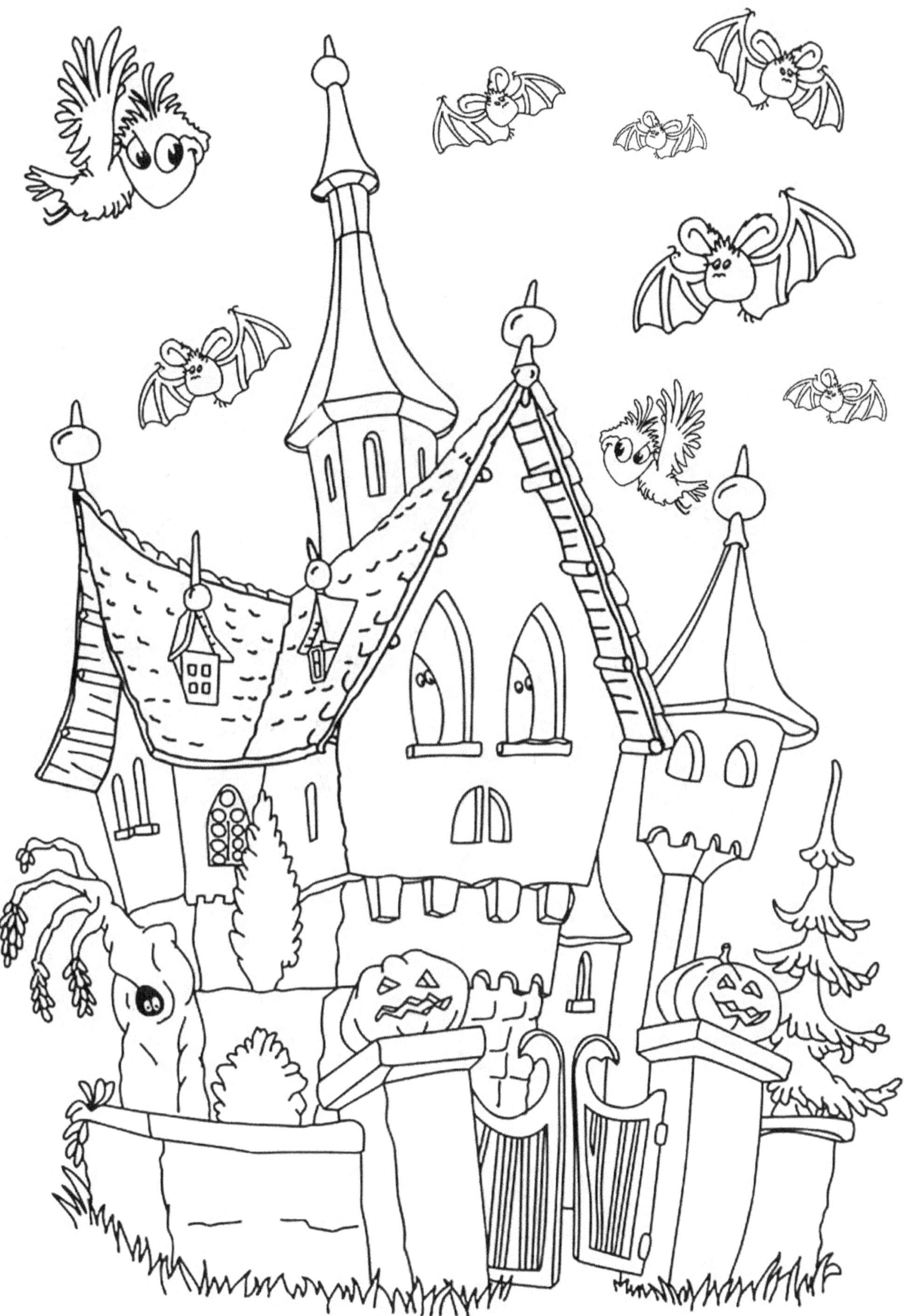

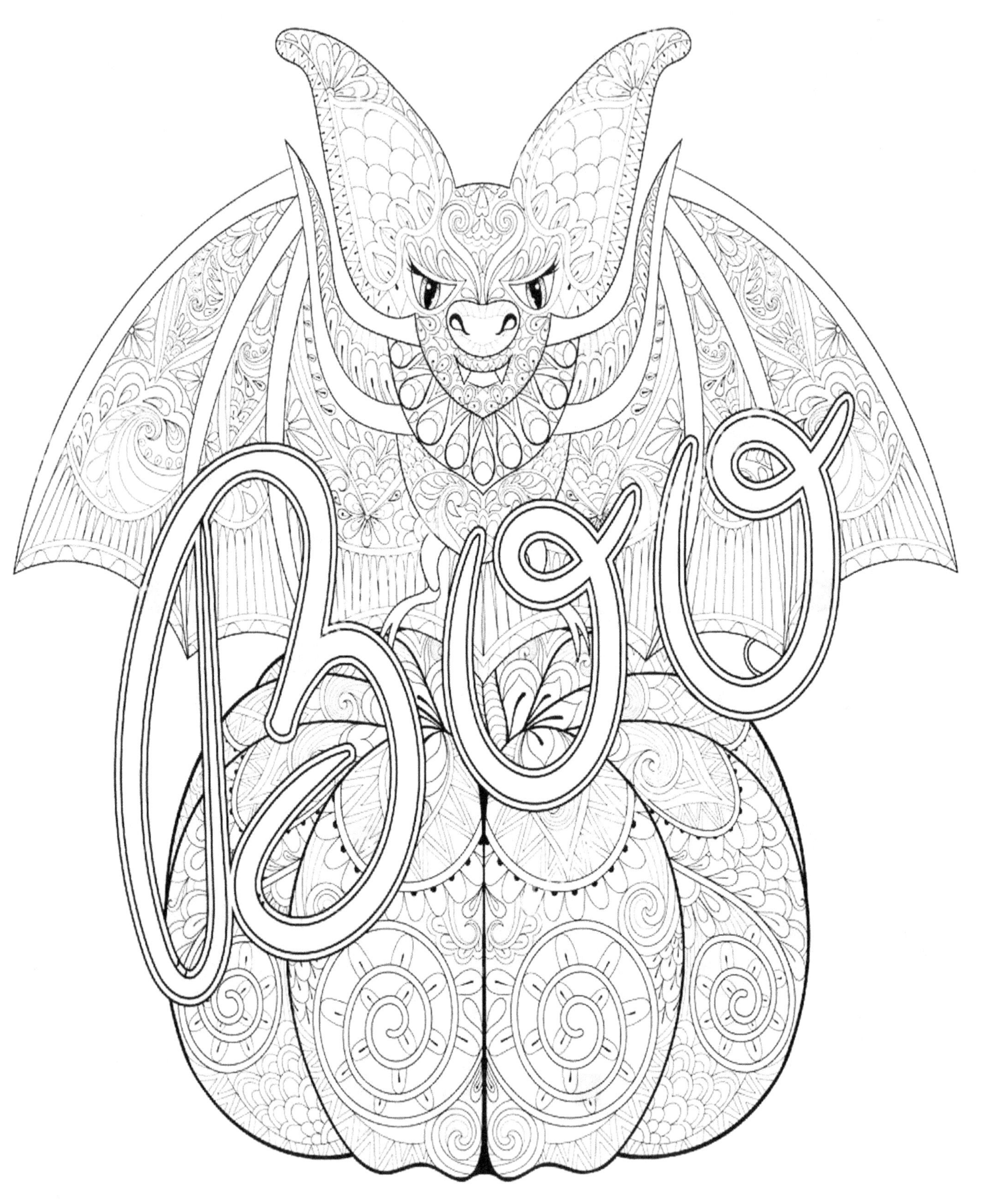

Boo

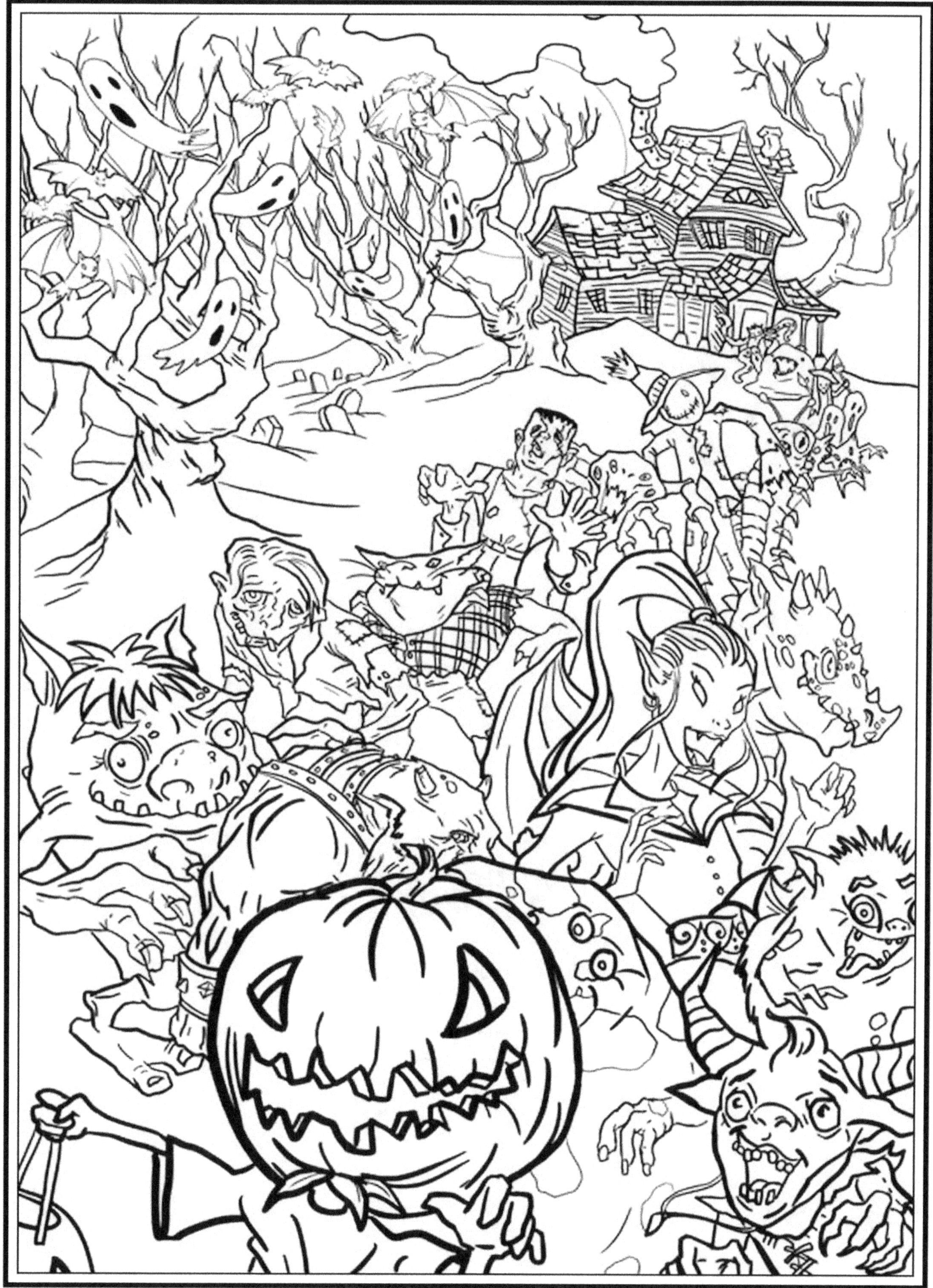

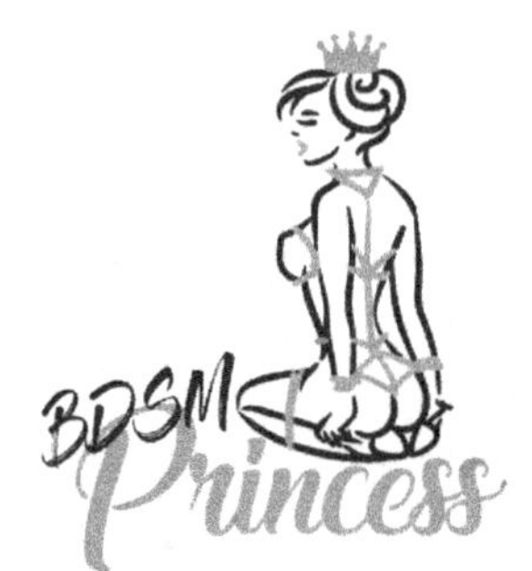

© 2019 BDSM Princess

Image Credits:
www.vecteezy.com
www.supercoloring.com